CW01271641

Inside .

Professional reflections of institutional life

Edited by

David Pilgrim

*Professor of Mental Health Policy, University of Central Lancashire
and
Consultant Clinical Psychologist, Lancashire Care NHS Trust*

*To Sue
with love
Dave*

Radcliffe Publishing
Oxford • New York

Radcliffe Publishing Ltd
18 Marcham Road
Abingdon
Oxon OX14 1AA
United Kingdom

www.radcliffe-oxford.com
Electronic catalogue and worldwide online ordering facility.

British Library Cataloguing in Publication Data

A catalogue record for this book is available from the British Library.

ISBN-13: 978 1 84619 106 0

Typeset by Phoenix Photosetting, Chatham, Kent
Printed and bound by TJI Digital, Padstow, Cornwall

Contents

Preface   iv
About the authors   v

1 Ashworth in context   1
   David Pilgrim

2 Pendulum   23
   Tom Mason

3 The disorder of things: an ethnographer's reflections from Park Lane   39
   in the 1980s and 1990s
   Joel Richman

4 Psychosocial interventions at Ashworth: an occupational delusion   59
   Mick McKeown

5 Listening to patients in 'Ashworth time'   81
   Carey Bamber

6 An account of the psychological team in Ashworth Women's Service   97
   Gill Aitken

7 Working in Ashworth Women's Service   119
   Lorna Jellicoe-Jones

8 Ashworth time   135
   Mark Chandley

Index   157

Preface

Ashworth, like all high-security hospitals, is isolated from the outside world most of the time. Members of staff come and go on a daily basis and a limited number of relatives, lawyers and external NHS staff visit patients behind its high outer walls. But outside of this limited interface with open society, the general public and the wider NHS workforce tend only to hear of the place under lurid circumstances or because of the occasional piece of leaked information about a particularly high-profile patient.

Because Ashworth is obscured from routine public gaze, any unknowing outsider will tend to invent their own view of what it contains. These disparate individual projections and assumptions are jolted by an episodic backdrop of scandal. Ashworth, like other high-security hospitals has had its fair share of scandals. These have emerged intermittently because the staff or the patients have behaved appallingly and have been exposed. Media revelations and official inquires then provide their particular account of these untoward events. All of the chapters in this book are in one sense a by-product of this recent history of publicised controversy.

Inquiries into staff or patient misbehaviour trigger media and official accounts, as well as more and more claims of clever management fixes. However, during varying periods of silence, public confessions of failure and immediate rhetorical flourishes about new beginnings, life behind the walls carries on. Little has been written about the routines in the hospital. This book offers those curious about the latter some insights from people who have known the hospital well and reflected honestly and intelligently about its organisational character.

Both critics and defenders agree that Ashworth is an extraordinary place. Because high-security hospitals are so unusual, we do need to understand as much as we can about them, beyond information gleaned from scandals and their aftermath. The following chapters start that task.

David Pilgrim
March 2007

About the authors

The editor

David Pilgrim is Professor of Mental Health Policy, University of Central Lancashire and Consultant Clinical Psychologist, Lancashire Care NHS Trust. He has worked between the NHS as a clinical psychologist and higher education as a mental health service researcher during his career. His books include *Key Concepts in Mental Health* (Sage, 2005) and *Mental Health Policy in Britain* (with Anne Rogers, Palgrave, 2003). His book, *A Sociology of Mental Health and Illness* (with Anne Rogers, Open University Press, 2005), won the British Medical Association's Medical Book Award for 2006.

The contributors

Tom Mason is Professor of Mental Health and Learning Disability at the University of Chester. He has worked and researched at Ashworth, Broadmoor and Rampton Hospitals and has spent 17 years in clinical practice and the remainder in research or academic posts. He was honoured with the International Association of Forensic Nurses Achievement Award in 1999. Tom has co-authored and co-edited 10 books and published over 70 journal articles. His books include *Seclusion and Mental Health: a break with the past* (with Ann Alty, Chapman Hall, 1994) and *Forensic Psychiatry: influences of evil* (Humana Press, 2005).

Joel Richman is Emeritus Professor of Medical Anthropology at Manchester Metropolitan University. He has co-authored a series of articles and conference presentations, focused on critical issues in the forensic domain generally and the 'special hospital' system in particular.

Mick McKeown is Principal Lecturer, Mental Health Nursing Research at the University of Central Lancashire. His publications include *Forensic Mental Health Care: a case study approach* (with co-editors Dave Mercer, Tom Mason and Ged McCann, Churchill Livingstone, 1999).

Carey Bamber is an ex-service user who was employed at Ashworth to develop a patient advocacy service. She is now a user consultant for the North West Care Service Improvement Partnership.

Gill Aitken is a freelance clinical psychologist who headed up the Psychological Service for women patients at Ashworth. Currently she works part-time as Lead Consultant, Women and Equalities, for the North West Care Service Improvement Partnership – Northwest Development Centre.

Lorna Jellicoe-Jones is Head of Psychological Services, Guild Lodge Secure Services, Lancashire Care NHS Trust. Her key areas of interest include Women's Service development and strategy. She worked as a clinical psychologist at Ashworth between 1997 and 2001.

Mark Chandley has been a staff nurse at Ashworth Hospital for the past twenty years. He is the co-author with Tom Mason of *Management of Violence and Aggression of Healthcare Workers* (Churchill Livingstone, 2005).

This book is dedicated to the memory of
Professor John Martin

Chapter 1

Ashworth in context

David Pilgrim

Introduction

Ashworth emerged from the amalgamation of the adjacent Moss Side and Park Lane Hospitals in 1990. When I worked as a psychologist at Moss Side in the mid-1980s, adverse reports about sister hospitals in the special hospital system (at Broadmoor and Rampton) were the talk of the wards and administration buildings. Yet to be scrutinised and yet to be criticised, the staff culture was divided between the complacent and the incredulous. In the first camp was the bulk of the nursing staff, championed by the Prison Officers' Association (POA). The POA considered that the regime was beyond reproach and that their members 'looked after some of the most dangerous people in Britain' (and variations on this refrain).

I was firmly in the incredulous camp. Still a young and relatively inexperienced psychologist I had worked for periods in an acute psychiatric setting and an out-patient psychotherapy clinic. I had come to expect a basic ethos of care towards patients (even if, in inpatient settings, that could be paternalistic). What I had not experienced, until going the Moss Side wards, was such stark old-fashioned institutionalisation and its Dickensian resonances for staff and patients alike. The nurses wore prison officers' uniforms, confusingly with a short white coat over the top. An older colleague, sympathising with my culture shock, suggested to me on several occasions that the problem with Moss Side, unlike Rampton and Broadmoor, was that it had *not* been the subject of an official inquiry. Neither of us realised at the time that his wish was soon to be granted, with explosive consequences.

The psychologists working in the hospital on the Moss Side site were often baffled and angry at what they encountered on a daily basis. We all witnessed a ward culture, which was anti-therapeutic and typically viewed patients as either enemies or as 'inmates' to be perennially distrusted. Foolishly, or bravely, I and other colleagues began to make a case for the closure of the hospital (Pilgrim, 1985; Pilgrim and Eisenberg, 1985). I received hate mail, and for a period was banned from the wards by the POA for my critical views. The experience was both distressing and eye opening. How could we be at the end of the 20th century and still find healthcare institutions with such authoritarian, undemocratic and anti-intellectual norms?

After three years I left, but never forgot the enormity of the place. Its physical spread was noteworthy (by now in most places, mainstream psychiatric wards were small corners of district general hospitals). But, far more importantly, the moral and political challenges of Ashworth – and by implication the other special hospitals – were gigantic. On the one hand, even stripped of the POA's overblown and demonising rhetoric about 'the most dangerous people in Britain', there were indeed many patients who had committed grievous acts of violence. The rapists, paedophiles and murderers were there in numbers (as they were and still are in the prison system). But there were many, particularly male, patients with learning disabilities, and those of the female side, who simply did not warrant high levels of security. Any intelligent lay person, let alone a trained mental health professional, could glean this once the patients' current risks and particular histories were examined.

In the case of those with learning disabilities, if the doors had been flung open, many of the patients were so disabled and institutionalised that they would have had neither the motivation nor the skill to leave or survive outside. As for the female patients, many were self-harming, with a high proportion of them being survivors of sexual and physical abuse in childhood. The ward staff often called women with learning disabilities the 'little ones', denoting their childlike status and to separate them conceptually from the brighter psychopathic patients, who were often held in suspicion and contempt. Both men and women with learning disabilities were sometimes in the hospital despite being non-offenders (they had been management problems in more open hospitals and had been transferred, many years previously).

In the midst of this mixed patient population there were many nurses who did all in their powers to act compassionately and supportively to their patients. Like all large institutions this was a place full of contradictions. A staff culture that was vast and impersonal on the whole, contained macho-authoritarian 'boot boys' with their far-right political sympathies at one end of the spectrum and heroic carers at the other. The latter stuck with the place far longer than I and many other disaffected souls managed.

Indeed I only realised afterwards that the majority of staff who stay at Ashworth for decades rather than a few years – maybe their whole working life in the case of many – were as often as trapped and alienated as the patients. Although the staff went home after their shift and took holidays, their world-view and existential horizons, like those of the patients, were chronically limited by the peculiar cultural forms that characterise a high-security hospital. Chapter 8 by Mark Chandley goes into this dimension of the institution in some detail.

In my experience at the time, the hospital was a place where paranoia, menace and mendacity were all around. Staff who might blow the whistle or not toe the party line would be ostracised or receive hate mail. I had to leave for the sake of my own sanity but the place stayed with me. Over the years I met up with old colleagues and some new to me who had worked or researched there but whom I had not encountered at the time. Each one told a version of a survivor story (as one might tell of surviving a war, a brutish boarding school or some other abnormally shocking period in one's life).

This book allows some of these people to tell their story. They are only a sample though. Many others could have told similar tales but wanted to leave Ashworth behind as a place best forgotten. Others I approached were still too close to the place or were ambivalent and erred on the side of caution. But before the rest of the chapters reveal a sample of perspectives borne of experience, I provide the reader new to the history of Ashworth with a context of understanding.

Victorian segregation

With an enlarging county asylum system in the mid-19th century (Rogers and Pilgrim, 2001), a subpopulation of criminal lunatics was identified that required more careful management and fail-safe sequestration. The first large and tailored institutional solution was Broadmoor Criminal Lunatic Asylum, which was opened in 1863. Its inmates were prisoners and some patient transfers from county asylums and Bethlem. They were criminals deemed to be not guilty due to insanity.

Prior to the Victorian asylum system, mad criminals, from the early 15th century had been incarcerated at home or in the local Bridewell (Allderidge, 1979). The Criminal Lunatics Act of 1800 had provided the legal framework to detain them. However, there was no designated and state-funded setting for disposal decisions by the courts about these doubly deviant individuals. Prior to the opening of Broadmoor, some parts of Bethlem Hospital in London had been set aside for this purpose by 1816 (O'Donoghue, 1914). The capacity of this wing of Bethlem was increased in 1838 but it was still insufficient in size for the population of criminal lunatics identified. As a consequence, the Home Office paid a private madhouse near Salisbury ('Fisherton House') to provide a special locked ward as an overspill for Bethlem in 1848.

By 1855, the lunacy commissioners who inspected the asylums were critical of the use of Bethlem, where criminal lunatics were placed in the same institution as non-offenders. By 1857 they had persuaded the government to build Broadmoor. This required a new Act for the custody and care of criminal lunatics, which was passed in 1860. Broadmoor started with 400 male and 100 female beds, with provision for later expansion. As Parker (1985) pointed out, this was already 100 fewer beds than first planned for, given the estimates of criminal lunatics dispersed across Bethlem and the wider county asylum system.

Moreover, overcrowding at Broadmoor was inevitable for another reason. From the outset it took prison transfers of dangerous and difficult-to-manage convicts, i.e. it did not solely absorb the criminal lunatic population from the asylums. Also, these two inmate populations were noted to be somewhat different. The asylum cases were more compliant and easy to manage (even though their index offence by definition had been violent in open society). By contrast, the convicts were incorrigible and this was seen to arise from their inherent nature and criminal lifestyle. At this point then the distinction between mentally ill offenders and psychopaths began to emerge.

Thus, the opening of Broadmoor was not a neat and simple solution, as it witnessed both capacity and management problems in relation to two different sorts of dangerousness. There was current or ongoing violence from some inmates, but others were no trouble (their *past* violence was the source of their incarceration). Also, the confluence of mental abnormality and criminality could still be found in a dispersed form across asylums, workhouses and parts of the penal system. By 1890 Broadmoor was completely full and so was granted more government support to expand. In 1900 work began on the Broadmoor extension but it was still insufficient, so pressure was eased further by the building of a new asylum adjacent to Parkhurst Prison in 1908 (Parkhurst Criminal Lunatic Asylum).

At the turn of the 20th century, legislation covering those with learning disabilities (the 1913 Mental Deficiency Act) provided further clarity about the institutional arrangements relating to dangerous inmates in the asylum system, to augment that given by the 1890 Lunacy Act. It soon became evident that some who were called 'idiots' or 'mentally defective' at the time were a management problem in more general facilities, and became candidates for secure institutions. This set a trend for the remaining part of the 20th century, in which people with learning disabilities, who were difficult to control, might be sent to Rampton, Moss Side or newly constructed medium-secure units.

The designation of Rampton as the main facility for these patients in 1920 allowed Moss Side for a while to be used for its original intention (as an 'epileptic colony'). However, during the 1920s the male wards at Rampton became overcrowded. In 1933, 50 male patients were transferred to Moss Side to ease congestion. Fifty-one female patients were transferred as well. However, this was not because of overcrowding in their Rampton wards. They were to be used as domestic labour in the kitchens and laundry of Moss Side. This practice was to diminish later as occupations departments absorbed those functions. It stopped completely when industrial action from the POA restricted patient movement in the hospital (Parker, 1985). Not only was this Rampton to Moss Side population more often about difficulties in managing those with learning disabilities, rather than their criminal pasts, the trend of containing non-criminality in Rampton and Moss Side was amplified by a viral epidemic.

The outbreak of encephalitis lethargica in the late 1920s led to a wide range of psychological abnormalities in its wake (Von Economo, 1931). Some children suffering from the virus were left with a form of brain damage that created both cognitive impairment and severe challenging behaviour. As a consequence, a trend was set of children being sent to what was to become the special hospital system. Rampton had its own dedicated facility for children until 1956, and it was only in 1980 that the last child was admitted to a special hospital.

By 1948, Broadmoor, Rampton and Moss Side had come under the control of the Ministry of Health. When plans for the NHS were formulated at the end of the Second World War, the asylum system for mental illness and mental handicap was omitted at first (with the intention of running it separately from the NHS) but at the last minute it was integrated (Webster, 1988). However, despite the new role for the Ministry of Health, the Home Secretary still retained control of admission and discharge to the three high-security hospitals. At this time, Rampton and Moss Side were designated as 'hospitals', and Broadmoor was now called 'Broadmoor Institution', rather than its original 'Criminal Lunatic Asylum'.

After the war, the Mental Health Act of 1930 was displaced by that of 1959. Under this new Act, the three institutions were to be set aside as a *system* of detention, designated under its section 97, for those deemed to require 'treatment under conditions of special security on account of their dangerous, violent or criminal propensity'. This set of options meant that it was lawful to continue to detain patients not sent from the criminal justice system (though the great bulk of 'disposals' were of this type).

This special hospital system thus retained different patient populations. Rampton for example still focused on those with learning disabilities, whereas

Broadmoor did not admit them. During the 1960s, Moss Side began to house a mixed population – male and female, offenders and some non-offenders, those with and without a learning disability, those with a diagnosis of mental illness and those deemed to be psychopathic. The development of Park Lane then added a layer of non-learning-disabled male patients when it opened.

Ashworth in the 20th century

The personal accounts offered in subsequent chapters emerged from a particularly troubled period in the past 20 years for Ashworth Hospital. But its oldest part had an unremarkable history, at least in relation to scandals. As was noted earlier, Moss Side Hospital was intended as an 'epileptic colony' just prior to the First World War but it was immediately used by the War Office as a military hospital for the treatment of 'shellshock' between 1914 and 1919. After the war the Lunacy Board regained control of it, and first Parkhurst prisoners and then Rampton Hospital patients were transferred there. The overspill function for Rampton was noted above, and during the Second World War more buildings were added and its bed capacity increased from 256 to 375.

Moss Side (and thus now Ashworth) was built about nine miles north of Liverpool, near the small town of Maghull, on a semi-rural edge of the Lancashire plain. The staff culture reflects this cusp position, with 'Scouse' and Lancashire accents mingling every day in the hospital. In 1974 Park Lane Hospital, essentially an overspill initiative to relieve overcrowding at Broadmoor, was opened using two old wards from Moss Side. The latter continued to function as a separate hospital, watching its shiny new neighbour expand to full site status by 1984.

Following the formation of Ashworth in 1990, the Moss Side buildings were closed in 1995. Park Lane had only contained male patients, but Moss Side had housed women for a number of years. With the amalgamation, the whole question of female patients in conditions of maximum security came to the fore (and is dealt with in Chapters 6 and 7 by Gill Aitken and Lorna Jellicoe-Jones).

By the 1980s large systemic changes were afoot in what was increasingly, if misleadingly, being called the 'mental health system' in developed countries. The reasons why large institutions lost credibility and momentum remain contested. Apart from claims about the putative 'pharmacological revolution', the costliness of the asylum system for the State (Offe, 1984) and the humanistic protest from 'anti-psychiatry', a series of hospital scandals came to the fore. (For a comparison of these arguments see Rogers and Pilgrim (2005)). Official inquiries into 'scandal hospitals' are described with great clarity in a book that appeared in the mid-1980s and was to be prescient about the Ashworth problem – John Martin's *Hospitals in Trouble* (Martin, 1984).

Martin reviewed all of the British scandal hospitals on record between 1965 and 1980. The last of these examined was the report on Rampton Hospital, where the mistreatment of patients was proven (Boynton, 1980). What was evident, when different hospitals were compared where a 'corruption of care' was there for all to see in the outcome of the investigations, was that large old institutions were good at warehousing chronic deviance but very poor at either rectifying it or attempting to do so respectfully and compassionately. Martin pointed out that these large institutions suffered from several layers of systemic isolation.

This emphasis on the systemic correctly draws our analytical attention away from the 'bad apple' theory of abuse and neglect. While morally suspect actors and acts may both be apparent at the endpoint of mistreatment, how do these acts come to emerge at all and why are their perpetrators given permission? Why is the run up to them not prevented? Why does the 'moral majority' not stop them happening? Martin argues that they emerge under conditions of multiple systemic isolation.

These large institutions are *physically isolated*. By definition they were built on the outskirts of towns or even in rural settings, reflecting the threat or offence their residents created for the wider moral order. They are also internally divided, leading to a fiefdom culture on particular wards. Such *cultural isolation* was endemic in all large institutions. Moreover, the staff is often *professionally isolated* – members of staff may work in one place all their lives and not be exposed to changing norms elsewhere in their profession.

The wards in these scandal hospitals were often nurse dominated, and medical visits were rare or set up in conditions not typical of daily routines. Thus Martin highlights the importance of *medical isolation*. Finally, the concentration of refractory cases means that these scandal hospitals had isolated chronic patient populations. This emphasis on *isolated and concentrated chronicity* means that the patients are easily disvalued and they offer little reward for staff effort.

Ashworth and other scandal hospitals after 1980

These systemic features were evident in all of the special hospitals. If Martin's overall thesis about multiple isolation was correct, then it was only a matter of time before all of them would manifest neglect or abuse towards patients. He was correct – between 1980 and 2000, Broadmoor, Rampton and Ashworth were all investigated and all were found lacking:

- *1980*: The Boynton Report (Boynton, 1980) confirmed the claims made by Yorkshire Television's *Secret Hospital* of brutality towards patients. Several nurses at Rampton were prosecuted and members of medical staff were relocated
- *1984*: The Ritchie Report into the death of Michael Martin at Broadmoor who died after being stripped, put into seclusion and injected with prn (when and if required) medication. He was the first of three black patients to die in conditions of restraint or seclusion at Broadmoor (*see* below), though the report did not identify explicit racism operating in this case (Special Hospital Service Authority (SHSA), 1993)
- *1988*: The Hospital Advisory Service delivered a report highly critical of the ward regimes at Broadmoor (NHS Hospital Advisory Service, 1988). The report argued that unless radical changes in the therapeutic ethos could be guaranteed then the viability of the institution was in question. Within months the government set up the SHSA to try to introduce general management principles into the special hospital system
- *1988/89*: another black patient, Joseph Watts, died at Broadmoor. Following a fracas with another patient, ward staff appeared with shields and helmets and entered his seclusion room. He was injected with a drug cocktail and within

minutes was dead. The report did not identify explicit racism but noted a lack of therapeutic aims, and isolation of the ward staff from the hospital's managers (SHSA, 1990)

- *1991*: the third black patient to die in similar circumstances was Orville Blackwood (SHSA, 1993). A pattern was now evident – being black and male brought with it substantial personal risks in secure settings (even if explicit personal racism was not evident to the investigators). Restraint and prn medication increase the risk of lethal cardiotoxic consequences. Seclusion solves an immediate problem of managing difficult behaviour for the staff, but it is not an act of care. Isolating any human being is the ultimate act of personal invalidation, because we are inherently social beings. Moreover, in hospitals rather than prisons there is a particular duty of care to ameliorate mental distress. Health care should not aggravate distress by denying the patient access to ordinary human contact. Solitary confinement inflicts this distress. Using the euphemism of 'seclusion' does not alter this fact

- *1992*: in the first of two major inquiries into the functioning of Ashworth Hospital, the Blom-Cooper Inquiry, like the Boynton committee over a decade earlier, emerged because of press scrutiny (Blom-Cooper *et al.*, 1992). The *Cutting Edge* documentary about Ashworth the previous year had exposed mistreatment in the hospital. Blom-Cooper investigated the implications of the programme's claims. For the first time an official inquiry recommended the closure of the hospital because of its incorrigible anti-therapeutic culture. By implication, following the reasoning of Martin cited above, the whole special hospital system should be closed.

This is not a comprehensive list of the inquiries directed at the special hospitals. Some previous reports had already established the risk of an anti-therapeutic ethos (e.g. Estimates Committee of the House of Commons, 1968; Elliott, 1973; NHS Hospital Advisory Service, 1975). Others focused on the risk of weak management or the tendency of management to become separated from ward culture (NHS Hospital Advisory Service, 1979). When the Health Advisory Service was invited to follow up the aftermath of the Blom-Cooper Inquiry in 1994, once again the risk of anti-therapeutic processes at ward level was highlighted, as were the problem of converting management principles into clinical norms. In particular, the difficulty ward staff had in formulating what their care plans meant for the habilitation or rehabilitation of patients in their care was highlighted (NHS Hospital Advisory Service, 1995).

Some inquiries have not been about mistreatment or the questionable capacity to develop humane therapeutic ward practices, but about patient risk. Some have focused on escapes from the system (from Broadmoor in 1981 and Rampton in 1994), and others about the smuggling of drugs and hard-core pornography into wards, and actual childhood molestation on site at Ashworth – the 'Fallon Inquiry' (Fallon *et al.*, 1999). This highlights that any institution that is set up to act as *both* a hospital *and* a prison can fail on either or both counts.

In the wake of the Fallon Inquiry, another one examining the risk of escapes from the high-security hospitals emphasised the need for more investment in structural security, rendering them even more penal in look and outlook, if the recommendations were to be accepted. The Tilt Report (Tilt *et al.*, 2000) offering the advice provoked some criticism from forensic psychiatrists about its anti-therapeutic implications (Exworthy and Gunn, 2003). In response, an Ashworth consultant highlighted the pendulum effect operating between Blom-Cooper and Fallon, which prompted Tilt. He cited the study of Rapoport (1960) in relation to alternating liberal disintegration and authoritarian reaction in complex institutions (Beales, 2004). (The use of the pendulum metaphor is pursued at some length in the Chapter 2 by Tom Mason.)

Thus, reducing risks in one direction inevitably raises them in the other; a sort of see-saw systemic effect. When a penal culture develops, it is *ipso facto* authoritarian, security obsessed and distrusting. But when risks are taken to take a credulous and trusting therapeutic attitude towards residents instead, then some of them will exploit the opportunity for personal gain. Blom-Cooper and Fallon, coming so close together in time, graphically highlighted this see-saw effect at Ashworth.

Despite Blom-Cooper focusing on the authoritarian aspects of Ashworth, and Fallon on the problems of the consequent over-liberal reaction in its wake, both argued for the closure of the hospital. The core consensus was that Ashworth was unmanageable and should not be allowed to continue to function. The NHS Health Advisory Service report in 1988 about Broadmoor had sent a similar signal. This focus on management was higher profile by the 1990s and can be contrasted with Martin's earlier focus (mid-1960s to 1980) on medical isolation. From the mid-1980s onwards, leadership in the healthcare system was less medically dominated and reflected a new policy (first supported by Margaret Thatcher) of a shift from administration to general management in the NHS (Rogers and Pilgrim, 1996).

The bulk of those entering this new managerial stratum were nurses. This posed, and still poses, a problem for all mental health services (not just in secure provision) because of the nursing workforce typically being both the source of problems and the source of the solution, when a clinical or organisational crisis occurs. This nurse domination means that other professions risk being marginalised. Also, any individual nurse who harbours doubts or criticisms tends to keep them private for fear of recriminations from colleagues. (Only one of the nurse contributors to this book is a staff member at the time of writing.) So maybe it was not surprising that none of the main witnesses in the Blom-Cooper Inquiry were nurses. They (the 'Ashworth Five') stepped forward instead from psychiatry, clinical psychology and social work.

By the time that the late 1990s arrived, the diagnosis offered about the special hospital system with its multifaceted malaise came from a newly installed top management team (Kaye and Franey, 1998). The latter authors, Chief Executives of the SHSA and Broadmoor Hospital respectively, were not willing to accept the nihilistic conclusion of Blom-Cooper. (Fallon had not reported at the time of their writing, with the same damning opinion.)

Blom-Cooper, in his covering letter to the Secretary of State for Health in July 1992, offered the view that he and his inquiry team questioned 'the need for the Special Hospitals within contemporary forensic psychiatric services'. In the text of the report we find the inquiry team:

> . . . felt that Ashworth and its problems belonged to a past era, and that the SHSA's attempts to transform an outmoded style of care into a centre of excellence of forensic psychiatric practice are doomed to failure . . .
>
> (Blom-Cooper *et al.*, 1992, p.164)

Thus Blom-Cooper was writing off not just Ashworth but the SHSA's attempts at, or rhetoric about, effective reform for the whole special hospital system. Not surprisingly, the new leadership team at the SHSA was not impressed. Kaye and Franey (1998) defiantly manifested the managerial equivalent of 'therapeutic optimism' and denied that the proposals for radical reform were a result of isolation or driven by external criticism. The message was that local managers were *already* able to appraise the gravity of the problem and, with the correct leadership, could continue to manage the hospitals successfully. A standard position of any new management regime faced with problems from the past is to argue that a plan is now 'in place' and corrective action is already in train.

This bullish optimism was not surprising. After all, managers are selected, at any level in an organisation but particularly at the top, because of their self-belief in the prospect of success. Without that confidence they would not aspire to acquire and enjoy their role. But this is also the very reason why judgements about the ultimate manageability of a system cannot reside with managers – it may be like inviting turkeys to vote for Christmas.

The context of Charles Kaye's appointment, as he admits (Kaye and Franey, 1998, p.35), was one of the highly critical NHS Hospital Advisory Service report on Broadmoor in 1988, which intimated its need to close. He was to be the chief executive of a new management body to get the special hospitals sorted out. Thus, because of its organisational separateness, the special hospital system began, for the first time, to experience general management principles. That first opportunity might also have been its last chance for managerial reform, as official reports were queuing up to argue for closure. The SHSA began to look like the last managerial throw of the dice to give the special hospitals a future.

All the evidence from Martin's work on scandal hospitals was that those who really exposed problems in a straightforward and honest way were either outside the system (for example the mass media) or newcomers to the system with little existential investment in it (new, especially junior, staff). Generally, the last to offer a realistic *public* appraisal of any organisation are those at the top of the political tree. Their job is to defend the sustainability of what they manage, not to argue for its demise or to give ammunition to those wanting this outcome. This understandable managerial desire for bushy-tailed optimism and 'good news management' is not a propitious starting point for the balanced appraisal of any organisation.

Nonetheless, maybe because all the facts pointed that way so incontrovertibly, Kaye and Franey began to concede an emerging alternative to the large special hospitals. They accepted the idea that the special hospital system might morph into dispersed units integrated with the regional secure system. (MIND, the largest mental health charity in England and a longstanding critic of the special hospitals, had been making this argument for at least 10 years.) The prospect of the special hospital system being broken up now seemed a real possibility, when its own senior managers were rehearsing scenarios about radical reform.

A relatively easy shift was to move control of the system from the central to the local state. This was a well-rehearsed political switch. From medieval times onwards, the responsibility for dangerous lunacy and idiocy had oscillated between central and local control. This shift back to the local state happened in two phases. First the SHSA gave way, in 1995, to the High Security Psychiatric Services Commissioning Board, with the latter now having a commissioning rather than a direct management role. Then, in 2002, the special hospital system was formally decommissioned, with the individual hospitals being incorporated into local NHS trusts. In the case of Ashworth it became part of Mersey Care NHS Trust.

Back to the future: Enoch Powell and medium security

The idea about dispersed smaller regional units reflecting different levels of security was not new and could be traced to the early 1960s by a working party ordered by the then Minister of Health, Enoch Powell. The working party argued that with the prospect of county asylum run-down, the role of secure facilities, including but not only the special hospitals, needed to be reviewed (Ministry of Health, 1961).

This began the argument for dispersed regional units, with varying levels of security, according to 'patient needs'. It can be noted here though that the latter has always been a mystification. Secure provision is offered primarily in response to the needs of others not patients. The psychiatric system has always been part of the coercive wing of the state to ensure the social control of some forms of deviance. In this sense mental health professionals have a dual loyalty – in one direction towards patients, and in another direction to third parties ('the public', the courts, the police, the penal system etc). The 'mental health industry' has always been about *both* humanitarianism *and* coercive social control (Scull, 1985).

High security brings this tension out most, and it is not surprising that, at a personal level, staff members often resolve the role conflict by straining in one direction or the other. They become *de facto* jailers or very pro-patients rights, and are frustrated by the constraints of security or they oscillate in their working lives between these positions. (I remember a judge, chairing one mental health tribunal I attended, who muttered that if he only listened to the predictably liberal views of clinical psychologists then he would be obliged to discharge each and every patient appealing to him, and the hospital would soon be empty.)

Despite the advocacy by Powell's working party of a new dispersed system by 1975, it did not materialise by that deadline (Bluglass, 1985). Indeed, during the 1960s, the lack of anything existing between the special hospitals on the one hand and the old county asylums on the other, with their attempts at offering an 'open-door policy', was a major problem in two senses.

First, it impeded the run-down of the asylums because they actually retained a security role, with some wards remaining locked for difficult-to-manage civil (i.e. non-offender) patients, who were sectioned under the Mental Health Act of 1959. Reactionary elements wanting to retain the old hospitals could point out that some inpatients still required locked containment (hence, conveniently for those opposed to hospital run-down, the whole asylum would need to survive). Second, the absence of what was to become known as 'medium security' meant that security was an all-or-none matter. A patient was either in an open hospital or they were detained as a high-risk criminal.

A particular problem (which remains today for many acute psychiatric wards) was that a minority of inpatients committed minor offences, when absconding, or created a public nuisance. It is not surprising that in addition to the search for medium security, eventually locked wards were to return in acute psychiatric units (euphemistically now called 'intensive care wards'). In the early 1970s, the government eventually began to concede the range of problems this gap between open wards and high security was creating, and set up two contemporaneous committees. The first examined the need for some non-offending patients to be contained in secure conditions – the 'Glancy Report' (Glancy Committee, 1974). The second was the report of the Butler Committee (1975) on mentally abnormal offenders.

From the outset, estimates of what was required were conservative. Around 2000 new beds, dispersed in small units, were suggested by Butler. Also, the notion of 'small' was always problematic. For example, Butler suggested 50 to 100 beds per new unit, but ones as large as 200 beds were not ruled out. When we consider that the Ashworth patient population has now shrunk to under 300 patients, then the gap in size between the current ex-special hospitals and the intended regional secure units (RSUs) may not be that great.

What the RSUs were to offer though was a range of new possibilities. First, there would be a fresh start – it would be a system untainted by past problems. Second, the role of the POA, with its authoritarian 'turnkey' culture, would be eliminated. RSUs might have a workforce with a nursing identity outweighing the jailer role, rather than vice versa. Third, they would be local services not national catchments. This provided advantages to both patients and their visiting relatives.

By the mid-1980s (over 20 years after Powell triggered their discussion), RSUs began to flicker into being. Though designated as 'medium security', escape from them was far from easy. However, their advantage was that an oppressive perimeter wall was not necessary (the looming penal symbol of Ashworth and the other high-security hospitals on approach).

Ashworth as historical product

Many of the current features of the high-security hospital system in England can be seen as a product of their history. For example, the mixing in the original Broadmoor population of residents who were there because of an historical act of violence in open society, and those who were still genuinely dangerous on a daily basis *inside* conditions of security remains today. A minority of patients in high and medium security are a genuine ongoing threat to those around them. But the majority of the patient population is not such a threat, as the contingencies that created their index offence are external to the institution. The two commonest examples of this are the sex offender for now denied access to potential victims, and the paranoid killer, whose mission is over now their victim is dead.

But the main point here is that the overblown POA rhetoric noted in the introduction does not really bear examination. When we now look at typical acute units in open hospitals, we find much riskier conditions. With lower staff–patient ratios, fewer options for risk management and more patients being admitted abusing (and sometimes trading in) substances, everyday ward life there is much more fraught for staff than in places like Ashworth.

Most patients in secure conditions, most of the time, are not troublesome or dangerous. (Whether or not they would remain in such a benign state in an open setting is of course a different matter.) Moreover, even when violence does erupt on wards – manifested by assaults on staff or other patients – it cannot automatically be attributed to the aggregate aggressive propensities of the population imported into the institution. Some of this violence accrues because of current contingent factors, such as boredom and the anomie created when detention is unending, as well as the peculiar group dynamics that emerge in closed, claustrophobic cultures. If patients have no hope of discharge, then what do they have to lose when venting their anger and frustration on any target, whether or not the latter morally deserves it? (The hostage incident reported by Cary Bamber in Chapter 5 is an example of this point.)

Complex closed systems tend to create paranoid destructive cultures in which, to use John Martin's phrase, the risk of the 'corruption of care' is ever-present. Martin's book remains a brilliant exposition about the dangers of large institutions for staff and residents alike. Isolation from wider society on a long-term basis creates systemic dangers that can exceed the aggregate danger of the offender-patients they contain. This is why concepts such as 'risk', 'threat', 'violence' and 'danger' quite legitimately have to be applied to the latter individuals with their offending histories. However, there should *also* be a parallel consideration of their meaning for all institutions that incarcerate those who wider society might distrust and disvalue. Hence the need to interrogate Ashworth and any other large institution that survives in what is now largely a post-institutional world.

What institutions like Ashworth and the other ex-special hospitals, with their dysfunctional histories, imply is a serious debate about what a democratic society is to do with those who are doubly deviant-mentally disordered offenders. A number of questions are begged in this debate. For example, what do we understand about this particular person's *prospective* threat to others? Does their *mental state* make a predictable contribution to that threat or is it irrelevant – might other variables have more predictive power? Are we detaining offenders *to punish them or to prevent further offending* (or both)?

Those who work both in secure psychiatric settings and in prisons know that honest answers to these questions lead to a variety of contingent answers. For example, many explosive domestic murders reflect a highly specific resolution to an existential challenge that will not repeat – the person had not been violent previously and is very unlikely to re-offend. The point then about detention seems to be a wholly one of punishment for the crime. It is not really one of risk management. In the case though of the incorrigible sex offender who has not killed a single victim, there is a much stronger case for prolonged, even lifelong detention, not as a punishment but as a preventative measure.

These examples show that temporary mental states and enduring personality features or sexual proclivities can shape our way of assessing risk to others in open systems. Moreover, that risk assessment remains more of an art than a science *because* outcomes in open systems are inherently unpredictable. Given this uncertainty, the current institutional arrangements we construct (mixing secure psychiatric facilities and penal arrangements) invite interrogation – are they effective at reversing deviance or do they simply keep it out of circulation for long periods? And are their corrective *or* preventative measures as humane as they could be?

There is certainly organisational confusion about where the state looks for answers. For example, some paedophiles and rapists are locked up in Ashworth or Broadmoor and not in a prison (and vice versa). The great bulk of sex offenders are in prison and most, because of the circular role of antisocial behaviour defining mental disorder (see pp. 17–18), could warrant a label of psychopathic disorder under current British law. At the same time, mental health professionals visiting prisons know that there are many mentally disordered offenders locked up in appalling conditions. This is particularly true for prisoners with learning disabilities and those who are currently psychotic.

The medium-security option invented in the 1970s by Butler and Glancy (Glancy Committee, 1974; Butler Committee, 1975) seemed to be one policy solution, but it has clearly not worked in relation to plugging the large gap between prison and maximum psychiatric security for two reasons. First, the bed capacity of the RSUs has not been large enough to absorb transfers from prisons, the ex-special hospitals and open psychiatric wards, as well as dealing with new referrals directly from the courts. Second, the RSUs have had little or nothing to offer those who are not deemed to be psychotic but who are sex offenders. And, like the special hospitals that preceded them, they also struggle to construct a credible treatment regime for those with *any* label of personality disorder (though they will admit these patients, whilst eschewing sex offenders). The RSUs, like their local open psychiatric partners in district general hospitals, have overwhelmingly become psychosis services.

If we take offenders with similar offending histories *and* similar psychiatric profiles there is no inevitable logic about their 'disposal', i.e. to prison or hospital. This would not matter if the rules and conditions about different places of detention were similar, but they are not. On the one hand it has been argued for many years that secure psychiatric settings tend to be much more humane environments because of greater resource allocation and their more medicalised ethos (Abramson, 1972). On the other hand, the psychiatric patient has to endure the challenge of open-ended detention, whereas the prisoner does not. Open-ended detention is not a humane process for anyone and creates demoralisation and deviance amplification (institutionalisation, skill loss and hospital-specific violence). It other words it has a demonstrable iatrogenic impact.

Moreover, turning to the healthcare sector as an organisational and political solution only ever deals with a proportion of offenders, given the high rates of mental disorder in the penal population. At the time when Abramson was arguing for more medicalised security, Scott (1974, 1975) was lamenting the plight of the large number of mentally disordered convicts always left behind in prisons. Around the same time, Monahan (1973) pointed out that the push for the psychiatrisation of offending rested on dubious grounds (*see* also Fennell, 1991).

Thus, it is it not self-evident that shifting the whole of the mentally disordered population over to the health service from the penal system would be either morally desirable or an organisationally effective basis for the *correction* of deviance. Nor would it necessarily lead to an aggregate or average mental health gain for the newly designated population. It might be more efficient though at risk *prevention*, because of its policy of open-ended detention.

Paradoxically, secure hospitals may be more efficient than prisons at prevention. We know this in relation to violent and sex offenders. These might leave prison quite quickly from a defined sentence spent without blemish inside. By contrast, similar offenders can spend many years in Ashworth with its option for caution. The defined sentence negates the prison system's responsibility for any re-offending, whereas secure hospitals could be found guilty of 'false-negative errors' in risk prediction. It is not surprising then that the opposite bias is evident most of the time.

The point here is that there is a debate to be had in society about the criminalisation or psychiatrisation of mentally disordered offenders. Moreover, this debate has to be informed not prejudice driven. The first body of knowledge to be considered should be about risk assessment of perpetrators in open and closed settings (not just the latter). The second is the risk assessment of the institutions themselves – not just their inmates. The third is about the cost–benefits of interventions. I use the latter term rather than 'treatment' (recognising a semantic conflation in the minds of many of us) deliberately.

For example, the so-called 'treatment' of sex offenders is essentially about the systematic application of techniques to allow offenders the opportunity to understand the consequences of their actions and the distorted ways they have rationalised them to date. This is a learning opportunity not a medical treatment. As for true medical treatments themselves, which remain largely medicinal in nature, cures are not on offer (hence terms like 'anti-psychotics' are misleading). Some people benefit some of the time from pharmacological solutions. Others remain unaffected or may fluctuate in their functioning, whether or not they are treated. They are sometimes called 'treatment resistant'.

What the penal and health systems have in common (reflected in the three bodies of knowledge just highlighted) is that they have converged about an *actuarial* approach. They are both now much more driven by risk calculations, whereas traditionally there has been a matter-of-fact confidence that to codify problems (in the prison or hospital) led to efficient expertise in 'rehabilitating' or 'treating' offenders (Armstrong, 2002). What the actuarial approach has done is open up tough questions about risk assessment, prediction and management.

The shift towards an actuarial approach in the past 30 years (in both hospital and penal settings) has highlighted the shortcomings of the medical jurisdiction over mental-disorder offenders. It has prompted (or been associated with) the problematisation of psychiatry as a legitimate agent of the state to deal with dangerousness. Once there was a taken-for-granted political assumption that a medical specialty does not just have *responsibility* for embodied mental abnormality, but is also competent about reversing that abnormality. Confidence has now been lost in this assumption from politicians, the public and even some in the profession of psychiatry itself (Bowden, 1985). To appraise the past, present and future legitimacy of troubled institutions like Ashworth, this wider discursive shift needs to be understood. It is no longer self-evident that mental health professions and hospitals are a solution. Maybe they are now part of the problem.

Bean (1985) points out that the confidence in a medical approach to the successful management of troublesome and dangerous individuals can be traced to the 1959 Mental Health Act and its preceding Royal Commission in 1957. The medical ideology it supported assumed that it was the legitimate role of psychiatry as a medical specialty to act on behalf of the state in two ways.

The first was role was one of *paternalism* (the legal concept of *parens patriae*). This is simple enough to understand under the ethical tradition of JS Mill and the exceptions he permitted (Gillon, 1991). Mill argued that all adults should always enjoy freedom, unless they broke the criminal law. However, for those whose mind was inadequate due to immaturity (children) or idiocy or lunacy, the state had a legal duty to offer them *protection*. The second delegation of state powers was in relation to *policing* the actions of those threatening society's moral order. Policing powers were also then delegated to the psychiatric wing of medicine (not just literally to the police force). The oft-used phrase 'risk to self or others' captures the two impulses of protecting patients and third parties and the role conflict it sets up for psychiatrists and other mental health professions.

This twin delegation has not always been comfortable for the psychiatric profession. Indeed it has been so discomforting that some have eschewed the coercive role altogether. An example here would be of the medical psychotherapist who will only work voluntarily with people with mental health problems. Others have objected to the jailer role expected of them for badness ('personality-disordered patients') but not madness (those with a 'severe mental illness') (Baker, 1992). The logic in the latter case is that doctors are trained to treat illness *and* they have an obligation or 'right' to treat it, even when the patient disagrees. What doctors are more ambivalent about is the same duty towards those who are not ill.

Psychiatry has had it both ways in this regard. As fecklessness, nuisance, immorality and amorality ('substance abuse' and 'personality disorder') were formally codified as forms of *mental disorder* by the profession during the 20th century, this would imply that doctors are now experts in diagnosing and treating them (Pilgrim and Rogers, 2003). But some psychiatrists want to opt out of that expectation or obligation – or they are ready to diagnose (the easy bit) and less ready to treat (the hard bit). At its most extreme, this culminates in troublesome patients in open psychiatric services being labelled as 'personality disordered' as a pretext not of treatment but of rejection from those services.

Others have rationalised their work as *only* being about medical paternalism, and have simply denied that psychiatry is about policing or rule enforcement at all. For example, the recent campaign of the Mental Health Alliance was joined by the Royal College of Psychiatrists. Its President, Mike Shooter, issued the following statement of concern about proposed legislation to replace the 1983 Mental Health Act:

> All of us have looked forward to new legislation to reflect changes in modern psychiatric practice. What we have got is a Public Order Bill that is ethically unacceptable and practically unworkable. We are proud to be joining every one who opposes it.
>
> (Pilgrim, 2007, p.91)

The implication of this statement is that psychiatry is not (or should not be) about 'public order'. However, ever since its inception as a profession in the mid-19th century, psychiatry has always been entangled with the coercive function of rule enforcement. By emphasising a 'duty of care' or a 'right to treat', the psychiatric profession has always been about public order, at least in part (Bean, 1980, 1985; Scull, 1985; cf. Ingleby, 1985).

Psychiatrists could only claim they were *not* agents of the state to maintain public order or they were *not* rule enforcers, if they all campaigned for the abolition of 'mental health' legislation and refused to work as a 'responsible medical officer' with explicit powers of compulsion. While ever the latter role exists and psychiatrists accept the status and salaries its state-delegated powers of compulsion afford, then they cannot reasonably complain of the public-order role expected of their profession.

These critical points about psychiatry can also be made about other mental health professions like nursing and clinical psychology. The whole 'psy complex', not just medicine, has ridden two horses – one about care and mental health gain and the other about social control on behalf of third parties. The psy complex has had to be involved in 'dirty work' on behalf of the state (Szasz, 1963; Emerson and Pollner, 1975).

Thus, if we are to unpick what Ashworth or any institution is about, on a range from pure voluntary contact through to coercive detention and treatment, we first must acknowledge that the two threads of paternalism and policing are woven into the fabric of professional action across the whole 'mental health system'. After that has been acknowledged and not mystified, by denying one thread or confusing one with the other, then we can begin to see why the actuarial approach to the *governance of dangerousness* has arisen and the logical, empirical and moral challenges it poses.

Ashworth as part of the governance of dangerousness

The clearest indication of the discursive shift towards dangerousness (rather than the notion of mental disorder *per se*) can be found in the British government's introduction of the notion of 'people with dangerous and severe personality disorder' (DSPD) (Department of Health/Home Office, 1999). The noteworthy aspect of this concept is that it was *politically invented* – it bears no relationship to the clinical discourse about 'personality disorder', which, by the way, itself is highly controversial (Manning, 2002; Pilgrim, 2001). Indeed, the government wanted to cut through professional equivocation about the label and its 'treatability' by insisting on using the new one of DSPD (Pilgrim, 2007). With this emphasis on the actuarial aspects of assessment and politically driven risk management strategies in mind, the current discursive context of Ashworth includes the following points of controversy:

- a *logical distinction between paternalistic care and control* can be made. If the two elements are conflated and not distinguished then we will not apply a clear and honest judgement about the effectiveness of care and control as separate enterprises. One of the problems for 'treatment in conditions of security' is that both enterprises are being attempted in unison, posing the next challenge
- *care and control may be synergistic on occasions but generally they are antagonistic*. On some occasions involuntary rules have to be applied as a precondition of effecting effective care (this can even be true in physical care, for example when treating an unconscious patient). But this is rare. Generally the more coercion is applied to others the less effective we can be in helping them because a helping relationship *ipso facto* has trust at its centre. This suggests that there are legitimate *a priori* doubts about the prospect of care when coercion is present (Pilgrim, 1988). Hence there are criticisms even of civil sections of the Mental Health Act, when patients are admitted and treated in open

psychiatric wards. When coercion is ever-present rather than episodic (i.e. in secure psychiatric settings), then these doubts amplify markedly

- *the field is plagued with tautology.* All functional mental disorders are defined in a tautological manner. For example, and with special relevance to arguments about offender patients, psychopathic disorder can be cited. Question: How do we know this man is a psychopath? Answer: Because he remorselessly raped many children. Question: Why did he rape the children? Answer: Because he is a psychopath. Tautological definitions of mental disorder are common and are to be enshrined in new British mental health law (Pilgrim, 2005)

- *the meaning and salience of dangerousness are socially constructed.* As Szasz (1963) pointed out, and many since have concurred, it is not dangerousness *per se* which is the issue, but the manner in which one is dangerous. Boxers, racing car drivers, mountaineers, military personnel (and their political masters) and astronauts all act in a more dangerous manner than others around them, but they are not coercively detained by the state. They are actually highly admired in society. Thus there is a variegated aesthetic of dangerousness – with some of it being liked, some of it being despised and some of it being tolerated as mundane or mildly amusing (e.g. being drunk). Public alarm and distaste tend to shape risk calculation and management rather than evidence or a strict cost–benefit analysis about *all* forms of danger in society. This means that risk calculations are as much about morality, politics and taste as they are about science (Radzinowicz and Hood, 1981). When it comes to assessing dangerousness, the large number of drunks responsible for road traffic accidents and domestic violence are recorded daily by the police. But the salience of their dangerousness is much less than that of mental-disordered offenders. The latter are small in number compared to our daily quota of drunks in every locality.

- *places not people often predict violence.* The whole logic of emphasising personal variables (whether these are clinical factors (symptoms) or personality factors) concentrates our actuarial efforts on people. However, where people are determines their actions as much as who they are (Hiday, 1995). This ecological point predicts the probability of both criminal features and mental state. Poor localities increase the risk of criminal action and criminal victimisation and they increase the risk of both first episodes and relapse in people with mental health problems. The relevance of this to us trying to assess and predict risk in secure settings is obvious – those settings do not have the same environmental contingencies as open society. When some spaces offer potential victims but others do not, then how can we make predictions from the latter to the former?

- *aggregate risk assessment is easier than risk prediction for an individual.* What the discursive shift to an actuarial model has pointed up is the serious challenge of predicting low-probability events in *individuals*. The mass murderer or the predatory paedophile spends most of their time doing unremarkable things like their non-offending neighbours. What we do know from the 'treatment' of sex offenders is that it is better to 'treat' than not 'treat' because the aggregate risk of re-offending is lower in the 'treated' group compared to untreated controls. However, what is not at all easy to predict is which *individuals* will or will not re-offend in either group (McGuire, 1995)

- *risk assessment does not always lead to accurate risk management.* So much of the activity of the psy complex in secure settings is about assessing risk. But risk assessment and risk management are not the same. The crudest default position is one of caution. This then leads to a tendency of false-positive bias – professionals do not get sacked for labelling a person dangerous when they are not, and an institution is not criticised for detaining them. If the reverse risk is taken, of releasing dangerous people erroneously judged in good faith to be safe, then professionals and institutions are criticised. Consequently, there is an understandable cultural tendency in secure hospitals to be risk averse, with all its human rights implications for unfairly detained patients (Blankstein, 1988)

- *clinical factors have been overvalued.* The state's reliance in the past on the role of clinicians as risk assessors and risk managers has led to a skewed discourse: clinical, particularly diagnostic, factors have been unduly emphasised. The shift to an actuarial approach has now clearly exposed this problem (Pilgrim and Rogers, 2003). For example, general diagnoses like 'schizophrenia' are useless predictors of violent action. Psychotic patients who do not abuse substances are not more dangerous than their neighbours in community settings (but the 'dual diagnosis' group is high risk) (Steadman *et al.*, 1998). The two individual diagnoses that are genuinely predictive of danger (substance abuse and antisocial personality disorder) are worth examining. In the case of substance misuse, all disinhibiting substances increase the risk in all those imbibing them, whether or not they and their actions are labelled psychiatrically. As noted earlier, most criminal acts under the influence of alcohol are committed by people with no formal diagnosis – the drunk driver or the abusive spouse are usually psychiatrically unremarkable. Substance misuse *as a diagnosis* is constructed or defined by a mixture of chronicity and help seeking. But it is with acute intoxication when violence typically spikes in probability and when 'substance misuse' is not usually diagnosed. Thus the formal diagnosis of substance abuse simply constructs a mentally disordered group out of a wide population which is also clearly dangerous but not, by and large, medically labelled. As for personality disorder, this is defined tautologically (see earlier point on tautology). Of course antisocial personalities are often violent; that is typically why they are called 'antisocial' in the first place. The best predictor of future behaviour is past behaviour in context. This truism applies to disordered as well as non-disordered action. Clinical factors add little to this general psychological rule.

Conclusion

The preceding text has provided a number of contextual points for reading the chapters to come. The organisational history of Ashworth was outlined. Its problems in part reflect its position in the state apparatus of social control in British society. The criticisms that accrued about it, leading to calls from many quarters for it to be closed down, are applicable to all large institutions, but especially ones containing and managing the double deviance of the mentally disordered offender. Thus these criticisms are equally applicable to Rampton or Broadmoor (or Carstairs State Hospital in Scotland).

The political need for, and standing of, these sorts of hospitals followed the trends of segregation and desegregation from the Victorian period onwards. By the middle of the 20th century they were at high risk of becoming scandalous – what John Martin called 'hospitals in trouble'. Multiple forms of systemic isolation ensured this outcome, with enough time, for all three institutions in the special hospital system. But even without scandals, the rationale for them weakened when it was obvious that their aspirations for cure and rehabilitation were blatantly floundering.

The consequent shift towards an actuarial approach to the governance of dangerousness exposed the many difficulties in relying on clinical expertise to solve political and moral challenges. The latter are mainly around what to do with people we do not like, especially when removing them from sight and trying to prevent their future antisocial actions. Locking them up indefinitely in an institution, which largely functions as a prison but is called a 'hospital', is a one-dimensional and unimaginative answer. It is costly in time and money, and constricts the lives for all residents (and staff too, albeit to less of an extent).

The chapters that follow are written by people who worked in Ashworth at a time when it was under double critical scrutiny. The institution seemed to be failing as a hospital *and* as a secure facility, as Blom-Cooper *et al.* (1992) and Fallon *et al.* (1999) respectively demonstrated. The reformist gesture of being brought under local control bought some time and temporary credibility. The loss of the female patients that was to ensue was another sign of reform, but it also implied that Ashworth was not a fit place for humane care. After all, in a post-feminist era at the turn of the 21st century, if Ashworth is not a fit place for women, why should it be a fit place for men? By the end of the book the reader no doubt will come to a personal view on the answer to this question.

References

Abramson M (1972) The criminalisation of mentally disordered behaviour: possible side effects of new mental health law. *Hospital and Community Psychiatry* **23**: 101–5.

Alldridge P (1979) Hospitals, madhouses and asylums: cycles in the care of the insane. *British Journal of Psychiatry* **34**: 321–34.

Armstrong S (2001) The emergence and implications of a mental health ethos in juvenile justice. *Sociology of Health and Illness* **24**: 599–620.

Baker E (1992) Dangerousness. The neglected gaoler: disorder and risk under the Mental Health Act 1983. *Journal of Forensic Psychiatry* **3**: 31–52.

Beales D (2004) Pendulum management in secure services. *British Journal of Psychiatry* **184**: 270–1.

Bean P (1980) *Compulsory Admissions to Mental Hospital*. London: Wiley.

Bean P (1985) Social control and social theory in secure accommodation. In: Gostin L (ed.) *Secure Provision: a review of special services for the mentally ill and mentally handicapped in England and Wales*. London: Tavistock, pp. 288–306.

Blankstein H (1988) Organisational approaches to institutional estimations of dangerousness in forensic psychiatric hospitals: a Dutch perspective. *International Journal of Law and Psychiatry* **11**: 341–5.

Blom-Cooper L, Brown M, Dolan R and Murphy E (1992) *Report of the Committee of Inquiry into Complaints about Ashworth Hospital*. Cm 2028. London: HMSO.

Bluglass R (1985) The development of regional secure units. In: Gostin L (ed.) *Secure Provision: a review of special services for the mentally ill and mentally handicapped in England and Wales*. London: Tavistock, pp. 153–75.

Bowden P (1985) Psychiatry and dangerousness: a counter renaissance? In: Gostin L (ed.) *Secure Provision: a review of special services for the mentally ill and mentally handicapped in England and Wales*. London: Tavistock, pp. 265–87.

Boynton J (1980) *Report of the Review of Rampton Hospital*. Cmnd 8073. London: HMSO.

Butler Committee (1975) *Report on the Committee of Mentally Disordered Offenders* Cmnd 6244. London: HMSO.

Department of Health/Home Office (1999) *People with Severe and Dangerous Personality Disorder*. London: Stationery Office.

Elliott JL (1973) *Report on the Organisational Problems and Staff Management Relationships of Rampton Hospital*. Unpublished NHS internal report.

Emerson RM and Pollner M (1975) Dirty work designations: their features and consequences in a psychiatric setting. *Social Problems* **3**: 243–54.

Estimates Committee of the House of Commons (1968) *Second Report: the special hospitals and the state hospital*. London: HMSO.

Exworthy T and Gunn J (2003) Taking another tilt at high secure hospitals. The Tilt Report and its consequences for secure psychiatric services. *British Journal of Psychiatry* **182**: 469–71.

Fallon P, Bluglass R, Edwards B and Daniels G (1999) *Report of the Committee of Inquiry into the Personality Disorder Unit, Ashworth Special Hospital*. Cm 4194. London: HMSO.

Fennell P (1991) Diversion of mentally disordered offenders from custody. *Criminal Law Review* **1**: 333–48.

Gillon R (1998) *Philosophical Medical Ethics*. London: Wiley.

Glancy Committee (1974) *Revised Report of the Working Party on Security in the NHS Psychiatric Hospitals*. London: HMSO.

Hiday V (1995) The social context of mental illness and violence. *Journal of Health and Social Behavior* **36**: 122–37.

Ingleby D (1985) Mental health and social order. In: Cohen S and Scull A (eds) *Social Control and the State*. Oxford: Basil Blackwell, pp. 141–90.

Kaye C and Franey A (eds) (1998) *Managing High Security Psychiatric Care*. London: Jessica Kingsley Publishers.

McGuire J (ed.) (1995) *What Works? Reducing re-offending, guidelines for research and practice*. London: Wiley.

Manning N (2002) Actor networks, policy networks and personality disorder. *Sociology of Health and Illness* **24**: 644–66.

Martin JP (1984) *Hospitals in Trouble*. Oxford: Basil Blackwell.

Ministry of Health (1961) *Special Hospitals: report of a working party*. London: HMSO.

Monahan J (1973) The psychiatrization of criminal behaviour: a reply. *Hospital and Community Psychiatry* **24**: 105–7.

NHS Hospital Advisory Service (1975) *Report on Broadmoor Hospital*. Sutton: NHS HAS.

NHS Hospital Advisory Service (1979) *Report on Broadmoor Hospital*. Sutton: NHS HAS.

NHS Hospital Advisory Service (1988) *Report on Broadmoor Hospital*. Sutton: NHS HAS.

NHS Hospital Advisory Service (1995) *With Care in Mind*. Sutton: NHS HAS.

O'Donoghue EG (1914) *The Story of Bethlem Hospital*. London: T Fisher Unwin.

Offe C (1984) *Contradictions of the Welfare State*. London: Hutchinson.

Parker E (1985) The development of secure provision. In: Gostin L (ed.) *Secure Provision: a review of special services for the mentally ill and mentally handicapped in England and Wales*. London: Tavistock, pp. 15–68.

Pilgrim D (1985) Whither the special hospitals? *OpenMind* **12**: 14.

Pilgrim D (1988) Psychotherapy in special hospitals – a case of failure to thrive. *Free Associations* **11**: 58–72.

Pilgrim D (2001) Disordered personalities and disordered concepts. *Journal of Mental Health* **10**: 253–66.

Pilgrim D (2005) Defining mental disorder: tautology in the service of sanity in British mental health legislation. *Journal of Mental Health* **14**: 435–43.

Pilgrim D (2007) New 'mental health' legislation for England and Wales: some aspects of consensus and conflict. *Journal of Social Policy* **36**: 1–17.

Pilgrim D and Eisenberg N (1985) Should special hospitals be phased out? *Bulletin of the British Psychological Society* **38**: 181–4.

Pilgrim D and Rogers A (2003) Mental disorder and violence: an empirical picture in context. *Journal of Mental Health* **12**: 7–18.

Radzinowicz L and Hood R (1981) Dangerousness and criminal justice: a few reflections. *Criminal Law Review* **3**: 756–61.

Rapoport R (1960) *Community as Doctor*. London: Social Science Paperbacks.

Rogers A and Pilgrim D (1996) *Mental Health Policy in Britain: a critical introduction*. Basingstoke: Macmillan.

Rogers A and Pilgrim D (2001) *Mental Health Policy in Britain* (2e). Basingstoke: Palgrave.

Rogers A and Pilgrim D (2005) *A Sociology of Mental Health and Illness*. Buckingham: Open University Press.

Scull A (1985) Humanitarianism or control? Some observations on the historiography of Anglo-American psychiatry. In: Cohen S and Scull A (eds) *Social Control and the State*. Oxford: Basil Blackwell, pp. 118–40.

Scott PD (1974) Solutions to the problem of the dangerous offender. *British Medical Journal* **4**: 640–1.

Scott PD (1975) *Has Psychiatry Failed in the Treatment of Offenders?* (The Fifth Denis Carroll Memorial Lecture). London: Institute for the Study and Treatment of Delinquency.

Special Hospital Service Authority (1990) *Inquiry into the Death of Joseph Watts*. London: SHSA.

Special Hospital Service Authority (1993) *Big Black and Dangerous? Report of the inquiry into the death in Broadmoor Hospital of Orville Blackwood and a review of the two other Afro-Caribbean patients*. London: SHSA

Steadman HJ, Mulvey EP, Monahan J *et al.* (1998) Violence by people discharged from acute psychiatric facilities and by others in the same neighbourhood. *Archives of General Psychiatry* **55**: 109.

Szasz TS (1963) *Law, Liberty and Psychiatry*. New York: Macmillan.

Tilt R, Perry B, Martin C *et al.* (2000) *Report of the Review of Security at the High Security Hospitals*. London: Department of Health.

Von Economo C (1931) *Encephalitis Lethargica: its sequelae and treatment*. Oxford: Oxford University Press.

Webster C (1988) *The Health Services Since the War. Volume I Problems of Health Care, The National Health Service Before 1957*. London: HMSO Books.

Chapter 2

Pendulum

Tom Mason

Introduction

Given the opportunity to reflect on my 30 years working in high-security psychiatric hospitals in the UK, and focusing specifically on the Ashworth experience, I approach the writing of this chapter in a reflective mood. This is necessary to recall the many memories available to me over this period of time. It is said that humans have the capacity to undertake reflexivity, which involves the bending of the mind back upon itself and thinking about thinking (Winter, 1989). It is a complex process in which the mind can recall a memory and hold itself up for examination through thinking about the feelings one had at the time of the event and the feeling one has now regarding those feelings. Thus, this 'enables us to reason and learn on the basis of past experience to stand outside that experience as it were and look at the present situation in the light of it' (Lee and Newby, 1987, p.317).

As I write these first few lines I am interested in what my mind will focus on when I come to write each section of my experience of working at Ashworth. Reflexivity is also concerned with holding up the situation under mental deliberation and analysing the courses of actions, causes and effects, and outcomes in relation to values, normative standards and codes of conduct, applicable in a particular context. In this spirit, I approach this chapter from two perspectives: first, from the perspective of the subjective self, an insider's view (that is from an internal reflective position), and second from the perspective of the more-or-less objective reality set in the context of the 'other'. I cannot guarantee that these two perspectives will be clearly delineated and kept separate, as one ultimately influences the other as a dynamic singular experience. Thus, the fusion of both perspectives will frequently be apparent.

Historical accounts are built on the shifting sands of perspectives involving ideologies, personal politics and stakeholder interests. But, so too, are the defences against those accounts. In this, rhyme, reason and rationales are offered in order to challenge and make sense of such histories. Different points of view exist because there are many vagaries to the functioning of humans, and when this human action is set within the structure and confines of a special hospital this cauldron produces a strange and amorphous brew. The latter is a cocktail of such potency that it inebriates the sober, dissolves the suppressing mechanisms and releases that which otherwise might be held in check. For example, it allows the mediocre to rise, the malevolent to surface and the weak to become powerful.

Wrapped up in mental health legislation, functioning as prisons, it is little wonder that these Disneylands of the damned are considered to be '. . . the last bastions of society's nightmare' (Richman and Mason, 1992, p.166).

Closed systems by nature, high-security hospitals have resisted many attempts to 'open' them up to external influences, from shocking TV documentaries to public inquiries, from restructuring and reorganisation to realignment of managerial and professional ethics, and from official reports calling for reform and liberalisation to official reports calling for increased safety and security. Yet, they have both resisted and persisted.

The experience of learning: rules, ropes, rehearsals and rites

Everyone who steps inside a special hospital as a professional for the first time will probably have some preconceived ideas, however accurate or inaccurate they may be, and a degree of trepidation as to what they will meet (for example, see early comments in Lorna Jellicoe-Jones' Chapter 7). What they are likely to see first may not be what they will eventually come to know: a totalising institution (Goffman, 1961) that is grounded in a dense macho culture (Mason and Mercer, 1998). These institutional arrangements and bullish ambience are based on the control of danger (patient behaviour, certain staff members), a tradition of experience (previous generations of staff and patients) and expert knowledge (skills of control). This perception of danger pervades the day-to-day business of the organisation. Experience is considered as high status both in terms of length and range of special hospital working, and equates with 'coming of age'. Expert knowledge is gained, not only experientially through the exercise in, and witnessing of, events, but also through storying, i.e. the recounting of 'experiences' in past events. Much of the early days is spent teaching the newcomer the rules of the organisation through stories of previous dangerous encounters that were overcome through skilled operations, difficult patients who were successfully managed by 'creative' staff, and violent encounters that were quashed through the power of staff groups. Stories contain much humour, usually at the patients' expense and targeted at the 'other' – that is, those on the outside of the nursing group including patients, other professions, management etc. They are largely around the topic of the dangerous individual, or situation, with the identification of a victim who is under serious threat, and usually conclude with how a nurse or group of nurses came to the rescue. This is the major theme of stories and jokes within Ashworth.

The stories are told and retold with embellishments until they take on a legendary form, becoming part of the folklore they are then, as important tribal accounts, passed on through cultural elders. They will be teeming with lessons to be learnt from the foolish actions of others who may have trusted an outsider, when trusting is only to be undertaken in each other inside a tightly closed group, i.e. nurses, doctors. These narratives are educational strategies by which traditional values are passed on to the next generation of practitioners and form the framework for distancing the culture from professional influences.

The stories are told to initiates as practising rites that must be adhered to, and forming the 'real' sphere of operations that challenge others' accounts. If others make professional suggestions to change or develop practice there is often an in-group response behind the scenes that 'they' are not living in the 'real world', which suggests that in a binary sense the suggested change is fantasy. Furthermore, each suggestion will be ridiculed by stories of past attempts that have failed, usually with many accompanying elements of danger, and conclusions involving the above rescue through the sensible reality of nursing staff. Thus, tradition equates with safety and security as 'real' and forms a grand cultural narrative that holds in abeyance the fantasy of change. This grand narrative is stronger and more all-encompassing than the grand narrative of psychiatry itself (see below).

The storying of cultural rules and regulations involves a close scrutiny of the listener. As an initial outsider, the newcomer is expected to respond to the stories with awe and without direct challenge or disbelief. They are watched closely to ensure that their passage from the out-group to the in-group is a safe one; that is, they are proving themselves not to be a 'spy' and are going to become a part of the cultural formation. Questions can be asked during the storying, but only questions of ignorance and not questions of dispute. The doctrine must be preserved intact. Therefore, the listener is observed for signs of acceptance and capitulation to the value framework, with increasingly 'risky' stories being told in response to an acceptable reaction from the newcomer. On the rare occasion that the newcomer rejects the stories by showing signs of disbelief, the 'risky' stories remain untold and the newcomer is considered 'unsafe'. In this situation they come to be viewed as 'rogue' and they rarely remain long in the institution.

A further role of the listener to the stories is as a witness. With each regaling, the listener is incorporated as a witness to the telling of the story, and in a sense becomes a witness to the events that are told. If these events are not challenged, and they rarely are, the listener is culturally absorbed as an 'accomplice' to the happenings within the story and as a member of the traditional group. This is similar to the witnessing of a real event as their experience in the institution unfolds and they feel unable to challenge the cultural response to it, which then embroils them as members of the cultural group.

For example, the consumption of patient food by staff was commonplace, despite the acknowledgement that it was not permitted. Hearing stories of the previous theft of patient food, which may have been grossly embellished, with humorous effect, engages the listener as a witness whose reaction is closely monitored to ensure a safe passage to the next stage, which involves the current practice of eating patient food. This is then sedimented through the witnessing of current staff partaking of patient food without challenge. Thus, the newcomer is absorbed into the cultural framework and becomes a full member of the in-group once they too have eaten the food.

This strategy of moving through storying, witnessing and practising is apparent throughout the institution in many areas of operations, though it may later become problematic as careers are advanced. For example, a nurse who becomes a manager may attempt to issue edicts relating to the impropriety of eating patients' food, only to be reminded that they were guilty of the habit when they were on the wards in the past.

Storying has (at least) one other aspect to it in relation to the cultural dimension of Ashworth – the listener as a potential focus of criticism within a story. The staff member is cautioned about being considered a part of the 'danger' or of being 'weak' within the anecdote. However, it is considered a high status to be the focus of the story if you are considered to be part of the 'rescue' or skilled expert in the control of 'danger'. Furthermore, in becoming a part of a cultural group, one becomes the focus of the story by association. For example, shift groups, wards and hospitals themselves can be seen as cultural formations and, thus, be the focus of stories. Stories of Ashworth are told in relation to Broadmoor and Rampton as culturally different hospitals, as are tales of high-dependency wards in relation to medium- or low-dependency wards within each hospital. This subgrouping can be continued down to shifts and individuals on a particular ward.

Cultural fusion: the death of ideology and the birth of a chimera

The amalgamation of Moss Side and Park Lane to form Ashworth was described by the editor in Chapter 1. Early recruitment for Park Lane emanated from the Broadmoor pool of staff. Thus, on Merseyside, alongside each other, were two special hospitals. One predominantly managed mentally ill offenders (real or potential) and the other people with learning disabilities who had interfaced with the law or who, less commonly, had proved to be unmanageable because of violent conduct in mainstream NHS care (real or potential danger). As Moss Side had been initially recruited from Rampton they functioned in a similar fashion. Park Lane, on the other hand, made a loud claim that they would not reproduce the culture of Broadmoor. I will consider later whether this claim was sustainable.

During the 1970s, while training as a registered nurse for the mentally handicapped at Moss Side Hospital, I observed the slow emergence of Park Lane, from portacabins, to the building of new wards and ultimately the encapsulation by the high surrounding 'beaked' wall. At the inception of Park Lane, with a few portacabins and a couple of borrowed ring-fenced wards from Moss Side, the early management of a half dozen or so staff was directly recruited from Broadmoor. The latter recruitment was presumably because it was considered the sister hospital, with Park Lane being built to relieve the overcrowding at this older institution.

As Park Lane grew, it recruited from a variety of sources, usually the wider NHS but also from overseas, as well as a few from within other special hospitals in England. Its managers boasted a new dynamic approach to the treatment of mentally ill offenders, with cutting edge therapeutic interventions, which followed a planned management strategy emphasising innovation, creativity and forward thinking. Both the custom-built hospital and the therapeutic approach were to be at the vanguard of professional development and considered to be the 'state of the art'.

As a young student I asked the then chief nursing officer what was needed to become a charge nurse at this new special hospital. He advised me to complete my training at Moss Side, undertake more training within the NHS, gain as much experience outside of the special hospital system as I could, and then apply to Park Lane in the future. I spent five years gaining various qualifications and experiences including one year as a staff nurse in Broadmoor. Following this I found myself entering the exciting new hospital, Park Lane, in 1984 on a six-month induction/probationary period.

On completion of my six-month probationary period I undertook an interview with the charge nurse during which I admitted that I was missing something about this new dynamic Park Lane hospital. He asked me to expand so I told him that I could not see any new dynamic pioneering interventions and asked him where they were taking place. I informed him that I had not noticed any new creative management strategies nor any cutting-edge therapeutic approaches. With a wry smile he leaned forward and said 'that is because there isn't any'. The organisation was chicanery.

I began to look more carefully and noticed some tell-tale signs. As indicated above, the then senior managers had predominantly been recruited and promoted from Broadmoor, and on moving up to Merseyside had photocopied all the policies and procedures from the old hospital. I noted that underneath the façade of modernity and progress, which simply involved a pendulum-like swing from the overt signs of Broadmoor, the policies and procedures were a simple replication with minor modifications and a change of logo. The pendulum swing simply veiled the public, politicians' and professions' peering gaze.

This mystification included Park Lane staff wearing lounge suits while Broadmoor had prison officer uniforms. There were no peaked caps at Park Lane, while Broadmoor insisted on them being carried if not worn. Multicoloured attire at Park Lane contrasted with the stark uniform black at Broadmoor. The pendulum swing also included the use of first name terms at Park Lane, while the use 'Mr' or 'Boss' was employed to address staff at Broadmoor. Various timetables for hygiene inspections and cleaning duties were the norm at Broadmoor, whereas patients were allowed to sit in squalor at Park Lane under the guise that this was a 'progressive experiment', and various 'tight' security procedures at Broadmoor were 'loosened' at the modern Park Lane.

In reality there appeared to be little vision, creative thinking, innovation, or forward planning at Park Lane, merely an automatic swing of the pendulum in the obvious direction denoted and predicted by gravity towards a binary trajectory. This was confirmed with numerous observations of policies and procedures that are the more discreet functioning properties of large organisations. I noted that on the security checks at the handover from shift to shift, the layout of the security items in the clinical room cupboards was identical between Broadmoor and Park Lane. This even extended to the old wooden encased institutional bath thermometer that lay in its box, unused and dry from year to year. It lay there (and probably still does) and was checked three times a day as a security item, 365 days a year. Its overt function (albeit unused) is the measurement of the patient's bath water temperature. However, its covert function is for management to defend the hospital in any future court hearing should a patient scald himself when bathing. As the written policy clearly states that the temperature of the water should be within clear parameters and checked by a member of staff on duty, this shifts the burden of culpability from the 'hospital' to the 'staff'.

In almost 30 years, across special hospitals, I have never seen that bath thermometer used for its defined purpose, nor have I ever used it myself. Ashworth Hospital managers were fond of producing these overtly harmless, but practically useless or practically impossible, policies. Their intention was to protect the hospital and themselves as managers against future criticism.

Another example should suffice. A patient attempted to escape by sellotaping under his scrotum a piece of glass, which was to be used as a weapon on a coach trip from the hospital. The brisk rub-down searches could not possibly reveal such weapons. Having failed in his attempt to escape, the searching staff were berated and a management dictate was issued to the effect that on all trips out of the hospital the patients' scrotums were to be lifted and searched. I requested that another matter be raised, and that was the question of serious allegations of sexual abuse! I have never seen a scrotum lifted to be searched nor did I ever do so myself.

The merging of cultures and the emergence of a 'monster'

In 1990 it was decided to merge Moss Side hospital with Park Lane hospital to create Ashworth. The name emerged from a competition set by the managers for patients; the winner thus had their preferred offering enshrined in history. At one level it seemed sensible, as both hospitals at the time used the same ancillary services, i.e. laundry, kitchens, portering etc. Importantly, they also shared housing sites and social club facilities. However, the merging of the two cultures was a different matter. Moss Side had the traditional special hospital trappings of prison officer uniform, being addressed as 'Boss', was grounded in order and control, and had a clearly defined set of disciplinary procedures for patients' transgressions against certain codes of conduct. Park Lane was as outlined above at that period in time. Throughout the 1970s and 1980s, while Park Lane was being constructed, these two cultures had fought battles to preserve their identities; Moss Side had an established one while Park Lane was attempting to develop theirs. Conflicts included heated debates and actual outbreaks of aggression in the shared staff social club. Boundaries were never totally delineated as there were emerging Park Lane staff who preferred the traditional approaches and there were a few Moss Side staff who welcomed a change of direction. But, by and large, the battle lines were clear enough.

Merging these two cultures was always going to be a difficult task. It was decided that with the creation of Ashworth, 'North' would represent the old Park Lane, and 'East and South' would indicate the Moss Side sites. At first, across-site working was difficult, particularly in view of the uniform issue, as North patients did not like the black prison officer uniform approach, and East and South did not appreciate the civilian attire for work. This was later resolved with the closure of the South site and a reduction in the East. Those staff remaining decided to come out of uniform and agreed to wear the civilian code of dress and work across the existing Ashworth locations.

This pushed both cultural groups into the melting pot. What emerged was a conflicting set of values, norms and codes of expected conduct from both staff and patients that largely remained unresolved. Both sets of values had to be enacted, sometimes as subterfuge, sometimes more overtly, depending on the audience at any given time. Sabotage on both sides became a favourite tactic in the battle for supremacy, and ridicule of each other became commonplace. The cultural densities were reinforced by an explosion in the number of nurse managers, consultants and advisors who insisted on change but without any strategic formulation. They were aiming to change what to what? At the time there were at least two cultural hospitals operating under one rubric but with competing values.

In this confused and confusing state of affairs the Blom-Cooper Inquiry (Blom-Cooper *et al.*, 1992) was launched as a result of serious allegations of abuse by staff at Ashworth. The nursing cultural groups were not the only factors in this, as we will see below, but both groups did have large roles to play in it. It appeared that the inquiry was originally launched against allegations emanating from the old Park Lane, and only later implicated the old Moss Side. However, this depiction, with hindsight, is a moot point.

During this period there was extensive reorganisation and restructuring. A series of replacement chief executives and management teams, as well as numerous 'expert' nurses, 'consultants' and 'product champions' arrived. Each surge of 'new blood' propelled the pendulum. All that was pre-Blom-Cooper was considered bad and, therefore, all that was post-Blom-Cooper must be good. Ashworth was now completely rudderless (a pendulum is not a compass). They came without navigational charts and quickly founded on the 'rocks'. Unfortunately, they abandoned ship to those that remained and left Ashworth Hospital adrift.

The Special Hospital Service Authority (SHSA, formed late in 1989) was in full flight by now. They had witnessed a strike at Ashworth, the Blom-Cooper Inquiry and (as yet to be discovered) the establishment of a paedophile ring on the wards serviced by the visiting of a young girl. Each chief executive and newly ensconced management team proclaimed what had gone before was now over. Things were about to change. They called for certain 'heads to roll', for a change of direction and for everyone to 'sing from the same hymn sheet'. Each senior management team remained aloof and distant from the workforce, rarely visiting the wards, and claiming to be 'strategic' rather than 'operational'. This left the wards isolated, distanced from management and in a precariously unaccountable state.

As was noted above this allowed the establishment of a paedophile ring on one of the wards, which was serviced by a young girl being brought in during visiting by an ex-patient. The Fallon Inquiry (Fallon *et al.*, 1999) that followed clearly identified that the wards had little higher management leadership. They lacked direction and the pendulum had swung too far towards liberalism (the source of the conditions permitting the establishment of the paedophile ring). I reiterate that everything pre-Blom-Cooper (Blom-Cooper *et al.*, 1992) was considered 'bad' and everything up to Fallon (Fallon *et al.*, 1999) was viewed as 'good'. Staff were punished or rewarded according to the prevailing views at the time, which clearly favoured liberalising patient care. Following the Fallon Report the organisation swung the pendulum now towards security, control and safety.

However, in all these swinging times, the notion of therapy was in short supply, unsurprisingly. I say 'unsurprisingly', as by this time I had witnessed the creation of a time-vacuum for the patients, who were locked within the confines of Ashworth with little or no therapeutic input. The filling of this time-vacuum was via occupation at workshops, recreation in the gym, swimming pool, squash courts, social events, sports and cinema. Menus and activities were fulsome during holiday periods and tolerable the rest of the time. Isolated pockets of attempts at a therapeutic input were ridiculed, undermined and sabotaged. Even other professional groups were either indifferent, disinclined or disillusioned. For those that did attempt an intervention, they were easily thwarted by the patients' dismissal during liberal times, and the institutional demands for the prioritising of security, safety and control when the pendulum was in the opposite direction. A few tried. However, it is always sad to witness someone's enthusiasm stifled in attempting 'something' even when one knows it is likely to be doomed to failure, for whatever reason.

Psychic prison: hostages to misfortune

In organisational analysis there are numerous metaphors that can be employed to bring into relief certain aspects of an institution. For example, Gareth Morgan (1987) identified organisations as 'brains', cultures, political systems, transformations and instruments of domination, amongst others. In this section I wish to deal with another of Morgan's metaphors for organisations and that is as psychic prisons. The functioning of Ashworth is based on the misapplication of both the law and psychiatry. First, its existence is premised on mental health legislation that can be employed to compulsorily detain patients for involuntary treatment. Compulsory detention certainly does take place within mental health legislation but as I noted above the application of treatment is at best sparse.

The usual strategy of chicanery is to proclaim that the Mental Health Act merely requires a prevention of deterioration, with the concomitant assertion that incarceration in Ashworth is doing just that. Declarations of 'milieu' therapy are no longer convincing, nor is the heavy reliance on the psychopharmaceutical complex (Kean, 2006). Thus, in the absence of effective therapies, mental health legislation is being abused. It is simply a cover for the indefinite detention of patients.

Second, Ashworth as a mental health institution is premised on the principles of psychiatry and psychology. Yet, other than the provision of explanatory frameworks for patient behaviour, theoretically interesting in itself, little is offered in terms of efficacious therapeutic interventions (other than milieu and medicine). Furthermore, what is offered for forensic patients remains largely unresearched, unproven and untested. The poor follow-up rates of released forensic patients are clear testimony to this. No causal relationship between mental disorder and crime has been clearly established, and the number of false positives and negatives remains alarming. Mental state is either an irrelevance to predicting dangerousness, or its contribution is small compared to other more powerful variables, such as male gender, low social class, young age, alcohol abuse and, of course, the most obvious one of past violent action. If all violent action was convincingly co-constituted with mental disorder then most prisoners, soldiers, gangsters and boxers should be put in hospital for treatment, but they are not.

That psychiatry claimed the 'dangerous individual' within its sphere of operations is well documented and will not be addressed here. Yet, questions remain as to why this profession should continue, in the face of such outstanding and long-lasting failure, to produce either a clear framework of research, a series of effective applications or an alternative interprofessional approach. This was raised throughout the 1990s at Ashworth with the resultant protection of professional power bases and hierarchical structures. At one point a chief executive wanted to dismiss all the psychiatrists that refused to change practice. She was very shortly removed from office and moved on to a better job in the World Health Organization. Global successful groups such as Microsoft, British Petroleum, MacDonalds and BT, protect and perpetuate their own interests, and forensic psychiatry is no exception. But how is this maintained at Ashworth?

It is maintained through an immense and elaborate chicanery, a sham of labyrinthine proportions based on a form of 'groupthink'. The belief system is so entrenched that no one within the group is able to produce a challenge to the existing power structure. Despite some having internal reservations they are reduced to silence due to the strength of faith in their doctrine. All are concerned that they will be excommunicated and isolated from the highly rewarding remuneration that undertaking this pretence brings (there are few wealthy heretics).

It is also maintained through the production of 'knowledgeable experts' and the creation of 'facts' concerning the notion of forensic 'science'. Interpretations offer the illusion of understanding and reductionist subcategorising to form nosological frameworks and produce the mendacity of efficacy. Research is espoused, conferences attended, papers presented, seminars conducted and workshops engaged, which produces a grand narrative of forensic discourse. This is extended to the general public through the values of 'a caring profession' working tirelessly in a hospital setting to cure the sick. Ashworth is juxtaposed with 'real' hospitals to assist vicarious images by association. Documentary 'evidence' is assembled through clinical notes, care programme approach, care planning, case conferences, patient care team meetings, forms for all occasions, medical records, archives, risk assessments, all manner of instruments for collecting data, projects, communication books, journals, academic textbooks, and so on. The overall result is a convincing endeavour that is ultimately defunct.

The result of this for nurses is that they too are caught up in the production of sophistry. There have been nursing approaches that have insisted on the adoption of models of nursing care, the insertion of the nursing process, care planning approaches, use of risk assessment procedures and the completion of an abundance of paperwork surrounding the patients' daily activities. Some nurses have emerged as 'expert script writers' (Richman, 1998) and are informally employed across wards to manufacture good written accounts of a patient's care in an academic style, referenced from the published literature and made to look and sound convincing for external scrutiny.

This is chicanery *par excellence*. Administration has increased, with the production of return rates for all types of patient behaviours, and the main focus on risk assessment and risk management within care planning and the care programme approach. At the end of each shift, the evidence of a 'good' day is the completion of all documentation, updated, signed and filed. This was colloquially known as 'having the job boxed off'. What the patient did was largely irrelevant as long as they did not cause problems.

This psychic prison traps both the patients and the staff, and both are sad and sorry hostages to a misfortune, which is not always of their making. The patients are trapped in a system that has an average length of stay of 7–8 years, with some spending decades within this confinement. The staff are largely viewed by external peers as second class professionals practising on the fringes, under a mainly custodial role, who function in their trapped state in a form of unconscious 'groupthink'. As Morgan (1987, p.203) put it: 'The metaphor of a psychic prison may overdramatize how we become trapped by favored ways of thinking. But it certainly does not overdramatize the way organizations and their members can become trapped by the unconscious'.

Management mayhem on 'Maggie's farm'

Organisations exist at two levels. First, there are the individuals that work in it. They operationalise practices according to the interpretation of policies and procedures, with this enactment made possible through the wielding of power. Second, they exist as an 'apparatus' of state power that performs the function of the governing body. As Foucault points out, this apparatus comprises 'a thoroughly heterogeneous ensemble consisting of discourses, institutions, architectural forms, regulatory decisions, laws, administrative measures, scientific statements and philosophical, moral and philanthropic propositions' (Foucault, 1980, p.146). Those that operate an organisation do so by the exercise of power through the relationships between these elements of the apparatus.

As Holmes and Federman (2006) describe it: 'The disciplinary technologies deployed in forensic psychiatric settings represent a continuation and intensification of what happens in "ordinary places", such as schools and homes' (p.19). In creating Ashworth, as indicated above, an organisation emerged, grounded in at least two cultural mosaics, with an amalgamation of differing management foci. One was based on the micro-functioning of a hospital on a day-to-day basis, in which smooth operations of patient control, little of note happening and 'nothing to report' were regarded in high esteem. The other viewed macro-operations in relation to wider psychiatry, an engagement with at least the notion of therapy and the production of documentary evidence in support of this as high status. There were as many tensions between these two cultural management groups as there were within the clinical staff working on the wards. Partisan policies were adopted, in which one group of managers favoured their own culturally determined ward-based staff, with the resultant exacerbation of internal conflicts. Sabotage and subterfuge became rampant as power politics were played out.

At this time the SHSA was attempting to create large-scale changes, on a number of fronts, and the drive to force Ashworth to have closer working ties with the mainstream NHS was underway. Many initiatives were discussed, but at the time failed to materialise, for example linking Ashworth with closer working ties to a university and the hospital becoming part of a wider NHS trust or becoming a trust in its own right (this ultimately becoming the case).

As was pointed out above, a series of calamities and new chief executives brought waves of new managers. One such 'tsunami' established psychometric testing on many nurses to establish their 'suitability' for ward management posts. Following yet another restructuring, a large number of G grade charge nurses were demoted, only to be usurped by their previous staff nurses. These demoted charge nurses became known as 'disgruntled Gs', as they kept their salaries but lost their power.

This dynamic on the ward was clearly untenable, with numerous conflicts, lethargy becoming rampant and newly promoted nurses becoming increasingly disillusioned and powerless. Sickness rates spiralled, and patients were largely left to their own devices, choosing to sleep late into the day and stay awake during the night watching TV. Managers were incapable of responding as they became more distanced from the clinical interface and made decisions without consultation. In trying to respond to developments in the wider NHS, Ashworth floundered amidst a sea of changes.

In an atmosphere of panic, Ashworth had no clear vision as to where it ought to go next. To the political development of, the mythical creation of the dangerous severe personality disorder (DSPD) and the suggested nonsensical mental health legislative changes, Ashworth expanded into this domain with the building of a Portmeirion-style 'village' unit, which was custom-built for such patients. Ashworth suddenly claimed to have created 'social therapy' for the DSPD and employed a number of so-called 'social therapists'. However, no one could actually identify exactly what these therapists ought to do beyond the activities of daily living, i.e. washing clothes and ironing (in fact, social therapy dates from the 1930s if anyone had bothered to look, and its therapeutic focus is anthropological).

This expensive 'white elephant' dissolved in an embarrassing fiasco, and other more credible national units took over the role of provider. Another grandiose scheme to emerge at the time was the idea of a 'forensic institute' at Ashworth Hospital, and hot debate ensued with a number of external academic institutions. Not-so-hushed promises of professorial chairs, senior posts, research funding and collaborative work were the talk of the day, with the resultant 'deals' being done on a 'you scratch my back and I'll . . .' basis. This exploded into a ferocious assessment of whose career was in the ascendancy and whose was in decline – and whose could be helped along in the appropriate direction. These expensive forays into cul-de-sacs were followed by rumours of shrinkage, closure of beds and even take-overs by the prison service. The ambience of Ashworth at the time was somewhat Monty Pythonesque.

Ashworth Hospital had become an embarrassing place to work. While, personally, I had tried to remain loyal to Ashworth (through Moss Side and Park Lane experiences), I now felt at my apogee to the organisation. I began to be ashamed of informing enquiring strangers about my place of employment. I tried to distance myself from such political games and kept a focus on my research programme with my professional colleagues. We kept publishing and funding ourselves at conferences, while others absorbed their time with the Foucauldian micro-politics of organisational life. We felt the sabotage of management strategies that attempted, some successfully others less so, to undermine the research process, to tamper with ethics committee members, to sterilise certain research programmes and publications and to issue threats of disciplinary action, litigation or termination of employment.

The highly acclaimed and respected academic professor of forensic psychology, who was director of research at the time, was undermined by an ambitious but less academically able psychiatrist who was given the power to do so by a weak acting chief executive. The result of this was that the director of research resigned his directorship, which enabled the psychiatrist to be ensconced into this post with, yet another, catastrophic effect. In a short space of time the research department was in tatters and the new (yes, another one) chief executive wound it up with the loss of contracts and high-calibre research staff. While my contract was safe, I decided that I no longer wished to be associated with Ashworth and the immoral behaviour of its management. I obtained employment elsewhere and I walked out to the tune of Bob Dylan's song in my ears, 'I ain't gonna work on Maggie's Farm no more'.

'Perfect' patients and 'problem' staff

At my interview, some 30 years ago, at a special hospital, the chief nursing officer at the time accepted my application with the words 'the patients won't give you any problems that you can't solve, but the staff? Well that's another matter'. I was not quite sure what he meant then; but I am now. Down my career in the special hospitals, and in particular Ashworth, where I spent the majority of that 30 years, I met and worked with some of the most industrious, caring and compassionate people who I have the highest respect for. They kept on trying even in the face of such tremendous adversity from many sources including management, professional bodies, certain patients and their family members.

Similarly, I have also met many patients who, despite their crimes and conditions, evoked my respect and highest regard, as human beings facing deep remorse and regret and who were eager for recovery. On occasions I have identified a small number of staff who ought to be inpatients and a number of patients who would have done well being members of staff. Such role reversals are humorously entertaining but are also inherently perturbing.

Patients who engage in dangerous behaviour towards others, whatever that be, may do so because they are mentally ill, brain damaged or because they are 'bad'. This latter term is usually applied to the psychopathically disordered or the personality disordered. We have long known that in psychiatric practice, including the forensic arena, such behaviour as, say, violence and aggression is not at the high levels that the general public believes it to be. However, when it happens we are not surprised at it, nor do we overly respond to it, as it is a 'natural' part of aberrant human behaviour. This is not to say that it is acceptable, but simply that it is understandable in the nature of things.

This was elucidated in a paper entitled 'Revisiting the nursing management of the psychopath' in which the authors suggest that staff should never be surprised at the behaviour that these patients exhibit (Moran and Mason, 1996). These authors argue that 'psychopaths by nature will manipulate their environment and others in it, generally more effectively than the rest of the population, including ourselves ... they are adept at mood swings from pleasantness to aggressiveness and appear happiest when causing chaos and confusion' (Moran and Mason, 1996, p.191). Although this may well fit an explanatory framework for a malfunctioning brain or the psychopathically disordered, what of the aberrant behaviour of a few staff who engage in chaotic and disruptive behaviour? Presumably they are not mentally ill, or brain damaged, but their actions are without doubt 'bad'. Staff motivations for such behaviours may well be located in numerous self-justifications but, notwithstanding the pain that they cause, this does not justify the ends.

Let me outline a few hypothetical cases. Would the action of a consultant psychiatrist who prescribes a series of electroconvulsive treatments for a psychopath in response to their accusations of not being treated therapeutically by him be considered bad? This is followed up by the consultant psychiatrist submitting a tribunal report to the effect that the patient was considered a paedophile, but no evidence for that was forthcoming. Would the psychologist who wished to pursue a personal relationship with a patient and release personal information regarding the staff on the ward be considered bad? Would the social worker who is supposed to go on a home assessment to prepare for the release of a patient, but who goes drinking at lunchtime and delays the release by several weeks be considered 'bad'? Would a manager's personal vendetta against a certain gay member of staff by continually blocking any chance of advancement be considered bad? What of the male medical director's sexual advances to junior female psychiatrists and their refusal resulting in the blocking of their careers? What of the consultant psychiatrist who treats compulsorily detained paedophiles in the UK and then visits foreign countries to engage in paedophilic behaviour? What of the incessant taunting of patients locked up for many years and their lack of opportunity for release thwarted due to fabricated reports? What of the female nurse who sleeps with the male patient? What of the allegations of physical, sexual and emotional abuse of patients by nurses?

How can we begin to unravel this complexity at an individual level? Is it the institution that facilitates these behaviours? Whose responsibility is it? Who should do what? It is these latter few questions that I wrestle with on reflection. When staff engage in behaviours that may be deemed bad, or at least stand in serious opposition to a moral code of conduct, what role did others play, including myself? It is relatively easy to state what a professional code of conduct would suggest should be undertaken but what happens in reality? Professional groups tend to bind together with 'whistleblowing' considered a negative reaction even in the face of governmental and organisational requests for staff to come forward when bad practice is encountered.

We are faced with the culturally dense formation outlined earlier, and the conflicts between traditional and professional codes of conduct. Whistleblowing in the special hospitals is a rare event, with those who undertake it tending to be hounded out of the organisation. Whistleblowers in Ashworth were regarded as self-centred individuals rather than having high professional accountability. They were ridiculed behind the scenes, even by the managers who officially supported them, and subtle mechanisms were employed to perpetuate the low status of the whistleblower through jokes and puns.

The power of this gallows humour is felt by many (myself included). Humour was a powerful mechanism employed by the Blom-Cooper Inquiry (Blom-Cooper *et al.*, 1992) against the staff giving evidence, as the transcripts clearly reveal. Had those giving evidence attempted to be humorous they would be swiftly rebuked as irreverent. It appears that we are left with the focus on role modelling, leading by example and rewarding appropriate behaviour. Such a social learning emphasis is easily negated though by its mirror image: there are plenty of staff role models manifesting immoral rather than virtuous staff conduct. The account I gave earlier about story telling as a process of induction and socialisation into historically determined cultural norms highlights this point.

Ashworth and its management of evil: hear no . . . , speak no . . . , see no . . .

Cradled in the discourse of scientism, Ashworth comforted itself with a denial of evil, despite the fact that a number of its psychiatrists attempted to amass the 'Madam Tussaud's' caseload of notorious criminals, presumably, to wallow in their infamy. Unable to deal with the social construction of evil, some shield themselves against it by hiding within the psychopharmaceutical complex (Kean, 2006) and ride in the wake of the global drug companies' profit margins.

Despite judges, jurors, media and the public at large having the capacity to understand evil, acknowledge it and manage it within everyday social spheres, others are disturbed by it, to the extent of denial. The question to be posed is 'is

Ashworth Hospital an evil organisation?'. The answer from Holmes and
Federman (2006) is 'only if it embraces the micro-politics of the apparatus of the
state; that includes the law and psychiatry. My answer is only if it continues to
refuse to listen to the voices of the critics, only if it refuses to hear . . . 'the silent
scream' (Mason and Mercer, 1998, p.1).

For too long, given its relatively short existence, Ashworth has spoken with a
voice that drowns out the views of others (for example those amassed in this
book). It has denied speech that it disagrees with. It embraces public relations
mechanisms that sterilise free speech, and although the signing of the Official
Secrets Act is no longer a requirement, Ashworth continues to be a closed institution, which defends its inner workings by secret stealth. Its tactics involve the
stifling of inner voices, the quashing of whistleblowers, the thwarting of external
agencies to scrutinise its practices, and the denial of researchers to engage in scientific enquiry.

For too long it has illicitly employed the official and appropriate channels of
committees to impede and obstruct attempts to prise the institution open to the
fresh air of scrutiny. For far too long it has spoken in corridors, manipulating in
its Machiavellian fashion, denigrating behind closed doors and destroying where
it cannot control. The question is 'is Ashworth based on the philosophy of
horror?'. For McKeown and Stowell-Smith (2006), the answer is 'only if it
refuses to open up its practices for scrutiny'. My answer is 'only if it declines to
speak; if it is characterised by a discourse of denial' (Mason et al., 2006).

It appears that Ashworth is more than content to gather up the images of evil in
order to medicalise its response to it, and does so through the state apparatus as
mentioned above (Foucault, 1980). It absorbs it through legislation, psychiatrisation and psychopharmacology, through its hidden but not invisible architecture by
'softening' the bars on the windows, deflecting the vision of visitors through land-
scaped flower beds, treed 'avenues' and statuesque sculptures, and through a vast
technology of industrial equipment and recreational facilities.

The extent to which these latter mechanisms of the apparatus are actually used
and benefited by the patient is highly questionable. However, they are most certainly employed by Ashworth in the constant 'tour of visitors' itinerary' to
provide an image of modernity to the medicalisation process. It also absorbs them
through the temporal timetabling of events through the markers of the day, the
daily indent on the week, the passing of the seasons and the yearly notch on the
calendar of patients' lives.

The impact on this Ashworth medicalisation of evil has been observed to
influence the focus of actual care planning, and the question is 'is Ashworth able
to see beyond its narrow, inward and blinkered focus? For Mason et al. (2006),
only if it lifts its head, takes off its blinkers and sees with a wider panoramic
vision. For La Caze (2006) the answer is only if it moves through a process of
forgiving evil and begs forgiveness for itself. My answer is 'no', because
Ashworth sees no hope.

On hope or no hope

Our history is replete with crises that occurred and catastrophes that transpired.
We only need to glance at this decade, which at the time of writing is only two-

thirds over, and note the 9/11 World Trade Buildings attack, Afghanistan, Iraq, the Indonesian tsunami, the Pakistan earthquake and the London bombings to note some serious calamities. During these times hope may fade but should never die. Hope dies last (Terkel, 2003). When these terrible events occur there is a clear emergency and services are swung into action; many times these actions are brave and save lives, but many times further damage is unwittingly caused and it is simply a matter of surviving the immediacy of the crisis. In the aftermath another focus takes over: one of short-term survival in which recuperation is a tentative thread on life. Following this is a stage of slow rebuild and reconstruction, with a taking stock of the events, an examination of our responses to it, our roles in it, and how we can improve our future. What these terrible events have in common is a grounding in hope.

Ashworth Hospital has had its relative calamities, certainly as far as a 'hospital' is concerned: the amalgamation of Moss Side and Park Lane, the Blom-Cooper Inquiry Report, the Fallon Report, the Tilt Report, deaths in custody, numerous reorganisations, restructuring and new management teams with their concomitant reshuffles, demotions and promotions, with rocketing staff sickness rates, prescriptions of Prozac rampant and early retirement packages being a keenly sought-after exit strategy. Despite a figure of nine chief executives in twelve years (or was it twelve chief executives in nine years?) attempting to give direction to Ashworth, it continued to be a severely demoralised, destabilised and destructive organisation. Little wonder that hope is a scarce commodity in this unhappy context.

I will finish this chapter with a reflection on the past and another on the future. Looking back, it has been both a vastly rewarding experience and a deeply frustrating one. Vastly rewarding because I have been taught a considerable amount by the patients, nursing staff and the many other disciplines that I have worked with. Some of the knowledge was good, some not so good, but it all contributed to the 'experience'. It was deeply frustrating because of the failure of this organisation to come to fruition.

The Ashworth experience has left me in both a positive frame of mind and a negative one. Positive because I met so many hard-working people attempting to do an extremely difficult job, with few resources, amidst constant pressure and with little support. Also positive because in the face of catastrophes the best of the human spirit rises (usually). However, I am also negative because I understand human nature and its pessimistic qualities. The egotistical arrogance, sexualised power, nepotistic favouritism, fear of scrutiny, the pleasure of control, the gratification in others' fear, the indulgence of authority, the shared laughter in the struggle of the underdog, and the satisfaction in their failure, and so on. It needs special people to overcome these negative aspects. I am not sure whether they currently exist at Ashworth. However, I do live in hope, which is why I will leave the final few words to others.

Ashworth Hospital is assumed to be a caring organisation that has the best interests of all those that fall within its sphere of operations, that is, both staff and patients, but probably in very different ways. Miller and Hood (2006), two US counsellors, work with clients who have experienced evil in its widest manifestation. They argue that 'to restore and maintain hope in oneself that can then be passed on to clients, the counsellor may need a repertoire of self-care options as well as a flexibility in trying different options to stay in balance physically, mentally and spiritually' (p.364).

They go on to suggest that those engaged in the care of others should accept that some stories are simply more difficult to hear than others, and that certain stories are fundamentally awful. Let us assume that Ashworth is a caring organisation but with some awful stories. If so, Ashworth should accept its own limitations and vulnerabilities and not expect to be so quickly accepted back into the fold of respected psychiatry and 'understand that a quick fix or even a foreseeable fix to such awfulness may not exist. Rather they may need to do what . . . [others have] . . . suggested for such situations, wait for a sense of hope to return' (Miller and Hood, 2006, p.364).

References

Blom-Cooper L, Brown M, Dolan R and Murphy E (1992) *Report of the Committee of Inquiry into Complaints about Ashworth Hospital.* Cm 2028. London: HMSO.

Fallon P, Bluglass R, Edwards B and Daniels G (1999) *Report of the Committee of Inquiry into the Personality Disorder Unit, Ashworth Special Hospital.* Cm 4194. London: Stationery Office.

Foucault M (1980) The eye of power. In: Gordon C (ed.) *Power/knowledge and Selected Interviews and Other Writings 1972–1977.* New York: Pantheon Books, pp. 146–65.

Goffman E (1961) *Asylums: essays on the social situation of mental patients and other inmates.* Garden City, NY: Doubleday.

Holmes D and Federman C (2006) Organizations as evil structures. In: Mason T (ed.) *Forensic Psychiatry: influences of evil.* Totowa, NJ: Humana Press, pp. 15–30.

Kean B (2006) The psychopharmaceutical complex. In: Mason T (ed.) *Forensic Psychiatry: influences of evil.* Totowa, NJ: Humana Press, pp. 31–66.

La Caze M (2006) Should radical evil be forgiven. In: Mason T (ed.) *Forensic Psychiatry: influences of evil.* Totowa, NJ: Humana Press, pp. 273–94.

Lee D and Newby H (1987) *The Problem of Sociology.* London: Hutchinson.

Mason T and Mercer D (1998) *Critical Perspectives in Forensic Care: inside out.* London: Macmillan.

Mason T, Richman J and Mercer D (2006) The influence of evil on forensic clinical practice. In: Mason T (ed.) *Forensic Psychiatry: influences of evil.* Totowa, NJ: Humana Press, pp. 327–54.

McKeown M and Stowell-Smith M (2006) The comforts of evil: dangerous personalities in high-security hospitals and the horror film. In: Mason T (ed.) *Forensic Psychiatry: influences of evil.* Totowa, NJ: Humana Press, pp. 109–34.

Miller G and Hood R (2006) Hope in the face of evil. In: Mason T (ed.) *Forensic Psychiatry: influences of evil.* Totowa, NJ: Humana Press, pp. 355–66.

Moran T and Mason T (1996) Revisiting the nursing management of the psychopath. *Journal of Psychiatric and Mental Health Nursing* **3**: 189–94.

Morgan G (1987) *Images of Organisation.* London: Sage.

Richman J and Mason T (1992) Quo vadis the special hospitals? In: Scott S, Williams G, Platt S and Thomas H (eds) *Private Risks and Public Dangers.* Aldershot: Avebury, pp. 150–67.

Richman J (1998) The ceremonial and moral order of a ward for psychopaths. In: Mason T and Mercer D (eds) *Critical Perspectives in Forensic Care: inside out.* London: Macmillan, pp. 146–70.

Terkel S (2003) *Hope Dies Last.* New York: WW Norton.

Winter R (1989) *Learning from Experience.* London: Falmer Press.

Chapter 3

The disorder of things: an ethnographer's reflections from Park Lane in the 1980s and 1990s

Joel Richman

> We have some of the most dangerous, crazy people here, you would never guess what they get up to . . . never turn your back on them. That's just the staff!
>
> (oft-repeated nursing joke)

Discovering the bastion of our nightmares

When the *chi* (life spirit) of research is much diminished with old age, when this ethnographer's body moves with a stumbling gait, then it is time for the 'confessional' (Van Maanen, 1988). Regurgitating past research to admire its qualities, or wishing that it had been done differently, come to the fore. Above all, setting the record 'straight' and repelling critics can become compulsive. Goffman, who surprisingly published nothing on doing field work, in a tape recorded talk to the 1974 Pacific Sociological Association Meeting, argued that you would not more than once or twice in a lifetime read your field notes. My field notes have constantly been an open vista, causing guilt over my lack of intervention in some of the ward scenarios I faithfully recorded, treating the latter 'neutrally' as 'critical incidents' although I was often witnessing patient degradation. The 'critical incident' has been captured now as a nursing tool, an aid to clinical practice (e.g. Dachelet *et al.*, 1981). I used it as a methodological device for opening up new layers of data not immediately recognisable in everyday activities. It was a new probe into the non-observable.

My research into Ashworth (at that time my location studied was the 'Park Lane' part) lasted over a decade. My initial research at Ashworth was oblique, a product of my secondment to the Cheadle Royal Psychiatric Hospital almost 30 miles away in Cheshire. Cheadle Royal was part private, dating back a couple of hundred years, treating many women whose professional husbands had company health insurance; the rest was NHS. One ward, Derby, where I was, treated anorexia nervosa. After resistance from some of Cheadle's medical staff, I was allowed to do ward ethnography. The NHS psychiatrists from south Manchester refused my access to their wards' patients. The argument was that ethnography was not 'scientific'. One argued though that if I wanted to take a pint of blood from his patients that was fine.

However, my study of Cheadle's psychiatric patients did not prepare me for what I was to experience initially on Ashworth's wards from 1985 onwards. I was then not too certain what the core of the forensic tradition was. Cheadle's psychiatrists regarded their counterparts in the special hospitals as the 'thumb screw type', not 'proper' psychiatrists, like themselves who were 'talking therapy' orientated. As a consequence of the merger between Cheadle's school of nursing and that of Park Lane, primarily due to the friendship of the two directors of nursing respectively, an 'unholy alliance' was forged between these two disparate hospitals. This institutional relationship enabled me to gain access to Ashworth. There, my research was mainly episodic (Olesen, 1990), spending blocks of the summer vacation ensconced within Ashworth's high walls, which rumour had it could not be scaled by the SAS. One persistent feature of Ashworth had been its 'Rebecca Myths' (Gouldner, 1954). After the Blom-Cooper Inquiry (Blom-Cooper et al., 1992), it even set up a telephone line to check out current rumours.

It is rare for texts to specify the researcher's motivation for initiating studies. Hammond's classic, *Sociologists at Work* (1964), remains exceptional within its genre. For example, Lipset's case study of the International Typographical Union, we discover, was generated because his father was a lifelong member. For me, Ashworth was a secret society. No ethnographer had penetrated this 'forbidden city', as total institution, and captured its secrets. My preference had always been for research fields which few sociologists had accessed, e.g. describing my previous research in the field of gynaecology as 'walking on the moon' (Richman, 1994).

My Ashworth studies formed a paternoster of disparate topics, influenced more by opportunism, personal interest and emerging themes; like the installation of ward managers after the Blom-Cooper (Blom-Cooper et al., 1992) recommendations to impose order on the runaway wards. I become aware that Ashworth staff denoted social epochs in terms of pre and post Blom-Cooper. With no norms of engagement in this secret place, my role varied and it was sometimes sponsored by sections of the hospital's power structure. Although the findings were useful to higher management and I did staff workshops (feedback sessions), I refused payment. I did accept hospitality of staff hospital accommodation (now abolished).

For much of the time I became like a war correspondent, presenting images of the exotic or unknown – standing at the front line, but often taking no action. As a consequence, today I still carry a heavy guilt. As Capa (a famous war photographer, especially from the Spanish Civil War) remarked: 'if the picture is no good, you are not close enough'. My urge to get the full story was unbounded. Consequently, both patients and staff regarded me as foolish for being sometimes isolated with triple murderers, gathering stories of ritual killings and not expressing astonishment when a patient explains that he knifed someone 'to see what would happen'. Many patients were taboo breakers; that is what made them so interesting.

I go on now to describe how my Ashworth research unfolded and what I found. This archaeological dig juxtaposes the *out there* with the here and the *past* becoming the present. During the research I came to view the special hospital as a 'bastion of our nightmares' (Richman and Mason, 1992).

Peripheral knowledge of Ashworth

During the 1980s, nursing education was undergoing radical reorganisation. The Cheadle Royal School opened in 1961, providing spacious residential accommodation for its mental health nurses. However, in the 1980s the syllabus expanded. Basically, the school became untenable, despite the mutual sharing of modules with other local schools. 'Project 2000' wanted more community nursing, more mature entrants, a broader common foundation year and courses for the upgrading of enrolled nurses. The government also wanted the closing down of the nursing schools attached to special hospitals, ideally as a means for changing its closed culture. In Nottinghamshire, Rampton opted to buy student places from a nursing school outside the special hospitals.

The Cheadle Royal and Park Lane schools adopted a radical solution for their mutual problems. They decided to create a new school of nursing, to be known as the Elizabeth Campbell (EC) school, named after a notable retired matron from Cheadle. The more humanistic nursing culture of Cheadle aspired to temper the more 'authoritarian' one at Park Lane. The Wheeler Report (unpublished) into the special hospitals' schools damned the latter for perpetuating a deleterious, nursing culture, which was considered to be divisive from the rest of the NHS. I was delighted to be able to research the unique EC school; this provided welcome breaks from Cheadle's wards, some dominated by therapies involving patient collages of their lives – full of middle class woes of unsuccessful holidays, uncaring husbands and children: the typical 'Mrs Hillside syndrome' replete with endless rounds of tea and cakes,

The merger generated numerous committees. The curriculum development meetings elaborated respective ward philosophies and teaching aims. It was noticeable how Park Lane staff differed in their presentations from Cheadle; everything was hinged to safety and security. Their ward staff were not up to date with much nursing development. One high-dependency ward at Park Lane claimed to be using the nursing process but allegedly it was 'adapted to fit into ward routine, yet still meet the needs of individual patients'. When I asked the relevant staff to explain this particular mixed model, there was an embarrassing silence. The strategic meetings, consisting of higher management (doctors absented themselves), team leaders and union representatives soon came to decisions. The new school's funding was to be split one-third from Cheadle and two-thirds from Park Lane. A new director of the EC school was to be appointed from outside. The dominant union on each site was to represent student nurses. I was accepted and recognised as the 'research observer' for the educational board, which was set up as the governing body for the EC School.

Come the morning for the English National Board (ENB) to validate the new merger, all were still stapling the new 'document' and correcting syllabi. Surprisingly, the new submission was 'validated', but with a long shopping list of amendments. Many syllabi had to be rewritten as the course was proceeding. Political will carried the day. The principal nurse in charge of the specials from the Department of Health regarded the EC as a major way forward. The ENB liked to think of itself, too, as *avant garde* in this matter.

The merger enabled me to cultivate a great range of personnel, especially involved in Park Lane. One of the government's representatives warned me about the entrenched power position of the Prison Officers' Association (POA), initially regarded by me as an unusual union for nurses. He told me how at one impasse in a national bargaining meeting a POA representative allegedly asked him which 'prison do you want next burning down'. Later, I was to recognise the POA power at Park Lane – resisting change by its appealing symbolically and practically to its high wall. I was soon immersed in staff's patient stories, in the Park Lane dining room, teaching site and the social club. I learned how Park Lane had got the 'best patients' from Broadmoor, but 'worse staff', when it was founded. How those patients always criticised the food for not including turnips, their favourite. How one day a patient knocked on the door of the ward office, carrying the door from his room, complaining that it had come off its hinges. This story and similar warned outsiders, like me, how physically powerful and danger-ous the patients were.

The merger enabled me to make my first penetration of Park Lane. Being the merger's 'official biographer' I wanted to survey staff attitudes to the merger, replicating the one I had done at Cheadle (Richman, 1987). Given permission to visit the wards and interview nurses, I picked up much valuable 'extra informa-tion' about the special hospitals. They often referred to the newly built Park Lane's distinctiveness from the 'county hospital'. The latter was an outdated term for the 'old big bins', often rurally situated, now gone: an indication of staff's parochialism. They regarded the special hospital as a career for life, with some staff related to each other. Summer was best, with its unlimited overtime, on top of the special hospital lead (equivalent of danger money, which all got irrespec-tively, e.g. office staff).

With opportunistic sampling, 47 Cheadle Royal and 50 Park Lane staff were interviewed, mostly nursing. Approximately two-thirds of both Park Lane and Cheadle Royal staff claimed to know some merger details. Twenty-eight per cent of Cheadle staff were worried that Park Lane would dilute their 'tradition'. Park Lane was especially ambivalent about the role of female learners. Some argued that they would 'normalise' patient settings: females were regarded as being better 'diffusers' of potential violence, but Park Lane respondents forcibly argued that female learners would 'not fit easily into the wards'. 'Girls' (such as those at Cheadle Royal) could be disruptive, forming attachments with patients, or being manipulated by scheming patients into such relationships, fragmenting the nursing team. (Similar male attachments were not considered.)

Park Lane staff expressed more concern about the increased work load, espe-cially over security that learners would cause if not key holders. Recruitment switched towards those straight from school, reducing the numbers of more 'mature' types that Park Lane staff preferred. 'Girls' straight from school would need more staff vigilance, and protection, signalling for me a paternalistic machismo culture. By contrast, more Cheadle respondents argued that the merger would make student nurses more 'flexible'.

Although the selection of student nurses was intended for the new EC school, *per se*, Park Lane staff designated their own 'Park Lane learners', a label main-tained all through their training. Legally, they were supposed to make their own choice of hospital when qualified. Those designated as Park Lane students, mainly male, received more advantageous expenses over the females.

In summary, the activities related to the education merger normalised my iden-tity concerning the special hospital. Being an observer (cum participant) enabled me to network in the ramifications of committees. I interviewed Ashworth staff on the wards, sending each a copy of the report's findings. I interviewed prospective nurse students to tease out their lay models of mental illness, following up students on their initial ward placements. I asked lecturing Ashworth staff about what they considered esoteric themes, like Foucault on mental illness. I demonstrated my academic credentials by writing an article attacking the new 'mysticism' of health quality assurance (Lees *et al.*, 1987), emphasising its 'misfit' with mental health problematics (the paper elevated the Cheadle Royal Director of Nursing to lead author). I hung around the Ashworth social club and was invited to participate in ritual storytelling, often 'humorous', about those with mental illness. (I recounted extreme stories about a psychotic psychiatrist admitted to Cheadle Royal and how the staff also had initial difficulties in recognising who was really the patient to be admitted from the accompanying group entering the hospital hallway). All these role settings made me conspicuous and dissipated my 'outsiderness' – I gained validation as a reliable person to be immersed in the secrets within Ashworth's walls.

All the media presentation of the hospital had been all bad news in the style of 'mad axe man lives a life of luxury'. Much revolved around Ian Brady, the notorious 'Moors murderer'. For example *The People* (13 September, 1987) ran the story: 'Monster cracks up as he clutches girl's hand for last time'; a Christine Hart, 23 years, sold the story that she believed she was the daughter of Brady. Later, I learned from patients that they objected to Park Lane being called 'Brady's hospital'. (Park Lane was the most expensive hospital; in the early 1990s each bed cost over £100 000 per year.)

The Yorkshire Television report on Rampton entitled the *Secret Hospital* had precipitated the Boynton Inquiry (1980) into patient ill-treatment. The post-inquiry new medical director had referred to the special hospitals as 'the garbage cans for society's problems'. Post-Boynton gave me my first major insights into the special hospitals, for example about the large number of patients inappropriately detained and waiting to move on and out. In the 10 years post-Boynton when Rampton's patients fell from over 1000 to 560, the 122 patients for transfer to open psychiatric hospitals remained the same. Such was the stigma of special hospital patients, even within NHS psychiatric circles. Such was the power of the POA that it refused to allow management to carry out initial investigations into allegations of mistreatment.

Thus, I did not adopt the direct route via formal channels and research proposals to gain access, as at Cheadle Royal, where I faced an ethics committee headed by a priest who asked me where I stood regarding the Helsinki Declaration of Human Rights, 1977. Cheadle's nursing director approached his counterpart, vouching for my usefulness in giving another view of the wards. I did not know at the time that two wards in particular, Arnold and Blake, (all the wards were named after English literary figures, which meant little or nothing to patients) were causing concern to managers at Park Lane.

The Park Lane nurse manager was receiving the 'appropriate documentation', but he suspected things were 'wrong' on these two particular wards. He adopted a patrimonial style of management and called a grand assembly of his ward team leaders to size me up. I made a short comment, saying that Ashworth was misunderstood, nothing of substance had been written and I was willing to learn. The questions were friendly and I was *in*. My security badge put me in the medical division (having a doctorate). I was inducted into key holding, by recognising the two major, ward entrance keys hidden in a pile of others; warned about 'security', shown patients' weapons like razor blades fixed in toothbrushes and poisonous substances secretly incubated, given the advice that if taken hostage I should fight to the end, because rape was common!

My initial research role could be described as 'collusive co-operation' (Pollner and Emerson, 1983). I was not 'just an observer' but dependent on many others: the chief nursing officer requiring a 'report'; the cohesive nursing teams considered me one of them; not least the patients to whom I signalled I was not really staff because of my cultivated lack of precision in opening doors in one movement, in a nurse-like manner. (I deliberately stood and puzzled about which key was to be inserted.) Leaving the ward with patients under escort I got mingled up with them, confusing the staff's tally. Everything was counted, down to the last teaspoon; anything missing required a thorough search of patients and their rooms.

In the field on Arnold and Blake

These two wards were known as the 'sink', 'punishment block', 'end of the line' and the 'pits'. They were a dumping ground for patients who had created 'incidents' elsewhere. The term 'incident' covered a range of behaviour, from refusing medication to attacking staff or killing another patient. Together the two wards were often called the 'compound' because they had their own wall, very much in the colonial tradition. Staff who worked there had a high reputation because of its 'difficult' inmates. Some were under long-term seclusion, for being very dangerous: one killed a member of the judiciary; another was a prolific rapist and strangler of passengers. The nursing team averaged 10 per ward (most wards had seven).

Although Goffman (Lofland, 1989, p.130) said that the 'first day you'll see more than you'll ever see again and the things that you won't see again. So for the first day you should take notes all the time!'. For me every day in Park Lane was a *first day*. At times I could not believe my eyes. I had been intellectually seduced (by radical psychiatry) into the proposition that mental illness was a 'myth'. My time in Cheadle reinforced this. Most women patients there were basically unhappy with their lives. In dramatic contrast, Arnold and Blake (A and B) were like I imagined Bedlam.

Some patients were banging their heads rhythmically against the bathroom doors. One was constantly drinking tap water. Some adopted different postures and stereotypes; one was drilling with military precision; another walked slowly in a circle with head bowed like a Capuchin monk in meditation. Others had their ears to the TV and radiators. Some were sitting with coats over their heads. But others were quite 'normal', drinking tea and smoking. Generally, the staff kept themselves isolated from patients both physically and psychologically. At meal and medication times, orders to queue were shouted. Seclusion patients were released sporadically onto the ward 'specialled' by three staff. It took me a couple of days to slip away from the staff and mingle. The most surprising thing was that 'obviously disturbed' patients were treated as 'normal' and expected to follow instructions.

Staff never debated among themselves the nature of mental illness. The nursing office did not contain text books or journals. Staff read the tabloid news-papers. The latter, intended for the ward, rarely reached the patients. Some staff domesticated the ward. For example, one team leader ambled around in old bed slippers and sloppy cardigan. Others brought their weekly washing onto the ward. Most did not bring their own food but ate the patients'. Faced with the latter, I was reluctant to join the norm and brought in my own food. To encour-age me to be one of them the staff gave my sandwiches in the refrigerator to a patient, in 'error'. One team leader used a nursing assistant as a personal chef and butler, cooking for the team. Occasionally 'guests' from other wards were invited to these staff meals. Each team had its own emblematic crockery. This commen-sality reflected each team's particular solidarity. One team did hill walking on its day off.

I was engaged in 12 hours a day ward observations, with at least 4 hours after-wards making field notes. After a week I was getting exhausted, frequently nodding off for naps in the staff room. It was not unusual for staff to take similar long breaks there. My theoretical problem was to try and make sense of this 'alien' world. Feeling more confident I broke away from the nursing group and talked to patients – an unusual activity. Despite the ward philosophy being replete with various nursing activities, I could not recognise any in the daily routines. Staff and patients talked briefly during patient-initiated activities: e.g. asking the staff for a 'light' for 'ciggies'; or requesting 'ciggies'/tobacco which staff held for them (patients usually rolled their own, being cheaper). Tobacco was a major source of ward conflict. Staff liked to ration patients' smokes, to last to the next weekly 'canteen' (hospital shop) day. Patients were not trusted with cigarette lighters, as some were arsonists. I remember the first conversation I tried to initiate, the patient interjected that 'it wasn't him that burned down the S Tees bus depot'.

The staff interpreted the water-drinker's excess to it being an illness symptom or being malicious to cause trouble for them. Nurses tend to countenance only two sorts of hypothesis – disvalued action as illness or as malice. It is either a 'symptom' or 'behaviour/personality'. Biographical or current situational factors are not considered to render action intelligible. This de-contextualised view is also found from psychiatrists in Ashworth, as I note later Excessive drinking disturbs the body's metabolic balance and it can induce coma by the dilution of sodium. The water drinker told me 'he didn't like himself or being here': the anthropo-logical implication possibly being water as a mechanism for identity transformation, a self-ritual to 'influence' events. The 'monk' told me the ward's central area was his church. Probing, he pointed to the ward's wooden beams having a 'cross design'. 'Soldier boy' explained that military drill kept him fit, if he was recalled to the military. One ex-Broadmoor patient (you could distinguish them by the manner they 'boxed' their beds) constantly rubbed his head to make a bald patch. He explained he did it to release 'radioactivity'. He suffered badly from voices. The analogy with trepanning to release evil spirits came to mind. Those with uncontrollable voices tried to keep them out by covering their heads with coats, or by covering the radiators, which were the 'transmitters'.

Patients, all regarded as dangerous/tainted, were herded together. Other wards let theirs filter back to their own bedrooms. A and B patients had no spatial opportunity to go 'off stage'; all were public people. Patients disliked each other. At meal times they gobbled food as fast as possible in the small dining room, some choking. Those sent to A and B as punishment strongly resisted contact with actively psychotic patients who 'talked rubbish'. The only way some patients could go 'off stage', achieving some protection of self and meaningful identity, was to do it *in their heads*. No one disturbed/challenged head bangers, water drinkers, monks, soldiers, members of the royal family or other famous persons or head coverers etc.

The system was inducing 'greater craziness'. Caudill (1958, p.11) aptly remarked, 'the patients' role in the psychiatric hospital is the least clear of all, except with his relations to his therapist'. But in Park Lane even the latter was not clear. It was common for some patients to have had no contact with a psychiatrist for 6 months. The adjunct to A and B was a handicraft centre. A and B patients were not regarded as 'adequate' to leave the wards and go to the hospital's rehabilitation centre for wood and iron work, painting, building and upholstery etc. Many of the articles could be bought for their own rooms or as family gifts. Nursing staff never participated with A and B patients; most were left with paper and pencil. Their 'contributions' were binned afterwards, further infantilising these patients. The highlight of the session was the tea and toast break. On sunny days patients were allowed on the grass outside the wards. Some threw themselves on the ground, arms stretched, facing the sun – like mentally ill patients did in Japan (Caudill, 1958) trying to make connections with nature.

A and B, like Park Lane in general, was governed by the 'three hospital system'. Each ward had three teams of nurses. Policy dictated that only one female nurse could be a member. (This caused problems when female learners went on to the wards, the qualified female had to move.) Each team had a distinctive nursing style, determined by the character and preferences of the team leader. The three teams, except for the 'rapid handover', never discussed common issues or adopted a consistent approach.

One 'young' team turned work into a 'play', often ridiculing patients' mannerisms, chasing them around the wards and playing mixed games of snooker. (Every ward was dominated by a full-size snooker table). Another team was completely aloof, a 'good' day being if they never had to talk to a patient. It was a serious offence under this team regime for a patient just to touch a nurse to gain attention. By contrast, another team has much physical contact, sometimes with 'mock combat'. Each team used to get patients to declare which was their favourite nursing team. Teams were engaged in their own rivalry. One acclaimed their superiority by releasing the five seclusion patients into the general ward area. The subsequent shift was 'horrified' and promptly locked them up again!

One afternoon I could just not watch a nurse put a patient through a public degradation ceremony for some minor spillage of tea, without comment. (Almost everyone was some type of ward cleaner.) The nurse had him on his knees and was repeatedly shouting: 'you are a cunt, what are you?'. The patient had to affirm. Patients were astonished at what I did. The team treated it as a joke. However, I was reined in.

I was given the official role of 'key man'. When a seclusion room was opened, the 'radio man' stands 10 yards away; the key man opens the door; then three staff rush in, expecting resistance if a sedating injection has to be given. (The seclusion room had a moulded bed and shuttered windows. Food is given on paper plates and cups.) Trouble is expected if nurses are seen to take off their watches. Claims for torn shirts and new watches were common in reports of incidents.

I also had to accompany the psychiatrist visiting seclusion patients. Doctors and others who are not ward based are always booked in as 'visitors'. The psychiatrist had problems with one patient who was asking for increased medication to reduce his visions. (Unlike voices, visions are a rare psychiatric symptom.) He was already on 360 mg of haloperidol and 1400 mg of chlorpromazine daily, and basically was trying to get the psychiatrist to kill him. The only control the patient could exert was about his existence (this and other cases are discussed in Mercer and Richman, 2006).

Dilemmas about dissemination

I did not rush into print with my A and B experience. I knew that eventually it could get into the public arena but my wife threatened to leave if it did. She could not understand anyone wanting to spend a whole summer with such 'disgusting people'. I could not 'neutralise' the impact of my fitting A and B into the literature on ward culture. The totalistic studies of Stanton and Schwartz (1954) only talked of patient loss of 'privacy'. Henry's (1958) ward as social laboratory would have made A and B look like ethology (the study of animals in their natural environment). Thrasher and Smith (1964) crudely used Merton's role set analysing 'gangs' and 'confidence cliques' on wards: my data lacked their precision, as I had not quantified rates of interaction. Moos and Hoots' (1968) ward atmosphere scales and Paul's staff-resident interaction chronograph (SRIC) was a complicated sociometric design which I could not provide with its 10 subscales of amorphous categories like 'involvement', 'spontaneity', 'autonomy' etc. Presenting papers (Richman, 1989) I homed in on the anthropological model of wards as clans, teams and lineages and patients' ritualised behaviour as strategies of magic, to handle uncertainty.

I delayed rushing into print because I wanted to continue with my research. I felt very privileged to be the 'first' to enter this closed society. However, I was compelled to give the nursing director a 'summary'. I made it verbal. However, he took extensive notes, which I assumed would have restricted circulation to the higher echelons. Inevitably they were leaked. I had named one nurse as being particularly 'dangerous'.

I named one patient who should never have been on Park Lane, let alone A and B. He was an example of the lack of assessment and moving on. The staff described him as 'the best kitchen boy they ever had'. Each plate was washed in 2 minutes 24 seconds. The staff had no replacement for him. (It was relevant that during a hospital outbreak of salmonella, A and B were clear.) There were other patients, too, who were caught in disputes between psychiatrists as to whose patients they were. I recommended that some team leaders be replaced, and they were. The initial feedback workshops on A and B were met first with great hostility. I had anonymous letters and phone calls saying that I had betrayed them.

In the workshops I tried to bring together psychiatry and anthropology. Caudill (1958) had made an early plea for 'clinical anthropology'. I argued that the A and B staff worked with the closed logic of Azande witchcraft (Evans-Pritchard, 1937): proof of dangerousness, the dominant ideology, anything chosen could be 'evidence'. Rosenhan (1973) and others have argued similarly that any feature of behaviour could be transposed into a mental illness symptom. But I also found myself defending the very nurses of whom I had been so critical. Nurses always complained that psychiatrists and other non-nursing clinical staff, like psychologists, were never around when an 'incident' occurred on the ward. They were accused of being away from Park Lane earning 'exorbitant' fees as expert witnesses etc. Also, to diagnose a patient or formulate their conduct in a one-off office situation is limiting.

Caldwell and Naismith (1989), psychiatrists, had published a de-contextualised ecology of violent incidents on A and B. Just as the nurses limited their interpretation of 'incidents' to madness or badness, these medical authors failed in their hermeneutic task. They failed to grasp that the highest number of incidents were in the day area with the amplification of surveillance and control and in seclusion, with staff provocation – a demonstration of masculinity and a display of power on both sides. That Sunday and Monday produced peaks was due to possible 'bad visits'. Patients become helpless spectators when news of family crises arrives via visitors. Also, tobacco on the ward runs out, with the addicts grubbing around for 'dimps' in ash trays or assaulting those not returning cigarette exchanges.

Surviving as a researcher after my leaked report

After the internally 'leaked report', I was a marked individual. Some advised me not to go back. Those 'betrayed' were cool towards me, making it known that they would do nothing if I was in danger. Others regarded me as a very powerful person who could make 'things happen'. I thrived on the challenge. Research at Park Lane had become addictive. I was 'intellectually' stronger. The initial notion of the bizarre had been neutralised and I could talk to others with familiarity about patients' nicknames, e.g. 'wolfie' (who howled when strangling others) and 'cyclops' (who had plucked out his eye). Being an alternative/reliable line of communication I had no difficulty returning. My agenda was clear: (a) to review A and B after reorganisation; (b) to research the admission ward, Tennyson; and (c) to research Forster ward, the most exceptional one in the hospital: a ward for young psychopaths which the patients 'controlled', having access to their own records etc. Many nurses were fearful of being sent there, where patients were even known to send food back to the hospital kitchen if it was 'substandard'.

In A and B, two nursing teams tried to 'deflect' me. One strategy was for me to spend most time formally teaching the nurse learners. It did provide opportunity to examine how they presented a patient history to the newly reorganised patient care team meetings (PCTMs). One went into the records and found the last one made over a year ago about patient X; this was primarily copied. This was standard practice encouraged by some staff. It made me more aware of how patients were 'frozen' in time, with one image or formulation being permanently recycled. The other strategy was to give me many notes written by patients describing how well they were doing on the ward. One two-page note ended 'Park Lane is a great place. There's a drop in centre where I can go and take the "mick" out of everyone and you can wear jeans to social evening with dirty old pullovers. I am in the *best place*. I must close now with fondest wishes to the *nice kind nurse*'!

My advice was accepted for allowing patients to leave the ward more often and meet other patients at the 'social' (where lemonade could be drunk). New rules had also been circulated that staff do not monopolise the snooker table. One patient's letter described Park Lane as a 'holiday camp', but a bit like being in the army.

Some team leaders had been replaced with younger staff. The first time I saw one was when he was on his knees scrubbing the bathroom floor with four other patients. He had bought scented soap for the patients. I spent an afternoon with him in the local supermarket buying food (cheaper than at the hospital shop) for a newly introduced Saturday barbeque. All the patients warmed to him. Seclusion had become the exception (except for those designated by the Home Office). The new team leaders managed to get education staff to come to the wards to develop literacy programmes.

Patients welcomed me, but had overly high expectations of my role. One patient, new to me, explained that he had been fitted up in prison. His offence concerned resisting arrest strongly, injuring police. A few weeks before his EDR (earliest date of release) from jail, prison officers 'topped up' his medication. He refused and was sent to Park Lane for compulsory medication. This was a strategy, I was to hear frequently, used by prison officers to give prisoners a more appropriate sentence than one given by the courts. He wanted me to take up his case.

Goffman (1968) aptly refers to the psychiatric referral passage as a 'web of conspiracy'. In the 'social', patients pointed out a large man, with another who was 'comforting' the gentle giant. I was told that he never 'killed the child'. The best I could say was that I would 'try'. Most killers I talked to admitted the offence. I discovered what I thought was a new phenomenon: murderers can grieve for those they killed. For a time on the wards I was shadowed by a patient, 'hindering' some of my conversations. He had taken it upon himself to 'look after me'. The patient underground network had heard of alleged threats towards me.

Tennyson ward was again totally different. The staff had been phoning prior to my visit, to remind me of my promised stay. I was sincerely welcomed; all staff wanted to brief me. They gave me complete access to the documentation. They took pride in their role of assessing new patients for Ashworth and the courts. They refused to have intellectually inadequate staff. Seclusion, considered a soft option for the patient to escape from their clinical gaze, was exceptional. Each patient presented a jigsaw challenge; realising the limitation of medical records, staff relished their role as clinical detectives. The nurses' first task was the 'entrance ritual'. Often, the police escorting new patients liked to frighten them with tales of 'two foot' syringes put into their backsides, while patients were being viciously held down and molested. The terrified patient was put at ease, uncuffed, greeted, joked with, given refreshments, shown around the ward facilities, then left to mingle with the other patients.

Tennyson patients were not allowed to go 'off' ward and meet established patients. Members of staff were critical of management policies: 'you rarely see the latter on this ward'. Park Lane, according to them, had too many staff misfits. It was almost impossible, for example, to dismiss an 'inadequate' nurse, because of the complexity of civil service employment conditions of service. Tennyson faced a major dilemma. As most wards had no vacancies, assessed patients could not be allocated. This was one example of organisational inefficiency.

Receiving regional secure units (RSUs) also had their own criteria as to which patient would be more appropriate for their regimes. Suspicious of Park Lane's patient evaluations they would re-assess the special hospital patient, change the drug regime – sometimes with severe consequences; then the patient was returned to Park Lane in a worse condition than in which he left. Tennyson's clinical aims were then distorted. The staff had many heated debates about their blocked patients: should they themselves start treatment regimes or reassess the long-term stayers? To keep up the patients' morale they increased their time in sport and exercise in the gym and pool. I was encouraged to spend more time talking with them. I made my first detailed history of a serial killer. He dressed in the manner in which he was to appear in court, and wanted my opinion of the impact. He wanted to be known as the 'man in black'.

Dealing with personality disorder

Forster ward was the creation of Dr Hunter (the acting medical director in 1988). The hospital policy towards personality disorder (PD) was one of equal misery – to disperse them so each ward would share their 'manipulative' behaviour. Park Lane's population was classified as 25% PD. Hunter wrote:

> . . . psychopathically disordered patients in particular get a raw therapeutic deal . . . tended to be left to one side, without a clear analysis of the genesis of their behavioural problems, let alone clearly defined treatment plans . . . in the hope of maturation . . . would benefit from *milieu therapy*.
>
> (Hunter, 1988, p.6)

Forster was set up for the younger patients; average age was 26 years, but the criteria had slipped, one was 39 years. Of the 24 patients, two had a psychotic disorder. It was rumoured that psychoticism 'frightened' the PD patients. The PD patients assigned to look after them only agreed if supplied with white coats! Forster ward was unique in Europe. It had many visitors to see the experience of congregating PD patients together. Often a patient was allowed to imitate a nurse and show visitors around. Forster patients allowed me in provided that I supplied them first with feedback. Dr Hunter, wanting ethnographic data for his conference paper, also sponsored me.

By the time I entered Forster I was well immersed into psychiatric literature, knowing that PD was an enigma or a highly contested form of mental disorder. Forster inmates traded on this uncertainty, PD being a member's classification device. As no one understood them, they were therefore a 'mystery'. This aura gave them a claim of superiority within Ashworth; nurses, at best, were their equals. They took stringent measures to keep 'undesirable' patients from visiting their ward in the evening. A great deal of their violence was 'normal' in the context of their traditional working class roots. Not relying on the police, disputes were settled in their 'own way', especially concerning the family.

PD patients had elaborate theories to explain their moral status. Some wrote elaborate accounts for me. One, hearing that he was likely to have his stay extended by a decade, explained that fate/some force in the universe had transformed him into the person he was and that he did not willingly murder. His interpretation was not of the order 'I was controlled by voices' (like psychotic patients) but more of a 'genetic cosmology', paralleling the Manichaean world view of 'special creation' – there being a predefining, separate force for evil (as well as goodness). Another wrote that 'time was a leviathan of emotions', overwhelming him: only a 'diluted' form of spiritualising (goodness) was able to 'filtrate' him. To him the 'real' psychopaths were serial killers, completely out of control. Two hours before rising in the morning he developed thoughts to systemise the world in his favour.

My initial understanding that PD patients had no capacity for moral reasoning was rudely shattered. The ward resembled a cross between a Jesuit seminary and a Rabbinical college (Talmud Torah). Any event could be transposed into a moral issue. Some nurses tried to avoid Forster because any action had to produce moral justifications. It was not enough to fall back on professional knowledge or status ('I am a nurse, therefore do what I expect'). The hospital rules came under the same strictures. In theory, the hospital timetables were supposed to apply to all wards, but Forster gave them ductility. Patients had amassed a great deal of organisational information, especially of staff wrongdoings. These recordings became the 'poker chips' for their bureaucratic games. Forster was the only ward where I saw staff ask patients if they could take a slice of bread from food patients' allocation.

I examined the patient's code in the manner of Wieder's (1974) convict code:

- Patients must not grass, but can have cross-over relations with staff. Some of the older nurses brought in fishing books for interested PD patients, sharing hobbies.
- Staff relations can be cultivated, provided there is a useful pay off – e.g. being able to use the office phone.
- Patients must maintain a high standard of body hygiene. PD patients cultivated 'muscular parades' – shorts and t-shirts as totemic displays, also indicating potential, physical power.
- Nurses must exhibit the highest moral standards. They were there for the patients' benefit and must be kept on their toes – being visible most of the time. Patients argued that if it was not for them, nurses would not earn such high salaries. If nurses were too long on their breaks, patients would hammer the radiators. Staff can only take patient food with their permission. Staff must participate fully in ward games. One nurse had his tie taken each session, frozen in the freezer and returned at the end of the shift.
- Patients must not debase the 'new leaf strategy' (Richman, 1997). In order for doctors to focus on them, especially before a review tribunal, patients would self-degrade – not getting out of bed, not keeping themselves or their room clean, taking on a 'depressed role'. With the established medical gaze, patients 'recover' and the 'progress' is recorded. However, if this strategy was overused it would be debased and so worthless.

The official rules of the 'unit' were few: acting out behaviour was tolerated as long as it did not involve physical violence. Patients took responsibility for their own treatment programme. Self-seclusion was forbidden. Newcomers were allowed active non-intervention, remaining aloof, until ready to participate in ward activities. All had access to their ward records and if disagreeing with any content could add a 'codicil'.

Forster was cleaved by contradictory discourses (*see* Table 3.1). For example, the nurse director was opposed to the ward, and considered that its freedoms undermined security, setting a bad example for the other wards. Nurses were forced into non-professional roles: to exist having to adopt surrogate kin roles, emphasising extra talents like being a storyteller or long-distance runner. Therapeutic assumptions were confronted by the patient code of 'not grassing'. Patients in general were ambivalent about 'therapy'. When they had adopted their own meaningful identity they did not want this transposed in 'therapy'. Therapy was a 'Catch 22'. If a patient revealed more than his index offence then he was more dangerous than supposed. If he did not participate, the professional assumption then became that he was 'concealing'; again making him 'more dangerous'. It was interesting that the Blom-Cooper Inquiry (Blom-Cooper *et al.*, 1992) called for more therapy, assuming this was both of proven effectiveness and invariably valued by patients.

Table 3.1 Contradictory discourses

Discourse	*Contradiction*
1 Medical/psychological investments	Nursing head's scepticism
2 Security	Liberalism
3 Bureaucratic routinisation	Ideographic, unique ward (unit)
4 PD discourse	Normality (i.e. crime)
5 Therapeutic assumptions: what is 'acting out'? what is 'coming forth'?	Mystery (lay beliefs)
6 Leeway function of rules	Consistent justice
7 Professionalisms	Surrogate roles: father, friend, brother, playmate, storyteller, played by nurses
8 Therapy revealment	Psychopaths' identity/maintenance Grassing and social distance

After I left Forster, a patient was killed. I never spotted the happening. On returning, no one would talk about it. I was left with a feeling that the killing was maybe delayed, because of my presence. Giving feedback I discussed some interactions I could not understand. One consisted of two young PD patients playfully sitting on the knee of a nurse starting a shift. I suggested it was compensatory behaviour for not having their own father, or practising their propensity for violence. It was none of these: the behaviour was a 'welcoming ritual' signalling that the new shift would have an easy time!

Effects of the Blom-Cooper Inquiry

The Blom-Cooper Inquiry (Blom-Cooper *et al.*, 1992) is now an important historical benchmark. I wanted to examine the aftermath of the inquiry. Little had been written about the after effects of inquiries compared to their detailed hindsight aspects (Martin, 1984). The inquiry had seismic effects. The acting medical director could not be found (the report had called him the 'invisible man'). The report gained credence as *ex cathedra* truth. Its erudition was buttressed by a flowing, academic style. The text was peppered with quotes from the pantheon of the greats. There were quotes from Lord Salmon's lecture at the Hebrew University in 1960 (hence its own in-house joke about the smoking of the Salmon letter (Blom-Cooper *et al.*, vol. 1, p.9). We also find others cited like Cervantes, Machiavelli, BF Skinner and the ubiquitous Goffman. The legal challenge by the POA that Blom-Cooper was biased was masterfully neutralised: patients with mental impairments, according to the expert witness Gudjonsson, were competent respondents. The report's metaphors were compelling, especially involving the rites of purification (Richman and Mercer, 2000): 'only when the wound is cleansed can the healing begin' (Blom-Cooper *et al.*, vol. 1, p.7). Members of staff who attacked their institution were 'canonised' as the 'Ashworth 5', purists. The inquiry ran twice as many focus groups as the earlier Woolf Inquiry (Home Office, 1991) into the Manchester prison disturbance.

Blom-Cooper made 90 recommendations. The new order (salvation) was to be achieved by the 'trinity' of a *new culture* (according patients full dignity), being *therapy orientated* (the assumption being that this reduces staff/patient violence) with purposeful *leadership* (as guardians of the new organisation). All those unrefined concepts became the new mantra of the hospital, with no guidance though about how ordinary life could be enjoyed or normal conduct demonstrated by patients in a reformed but still closed institution. The latter had anticipated the Blom-Cooper findings by the prior installation of new ward managers to synthesise their team's input, bridging, hopefully, the gap between the wards and the rest of the higher management group.

I researched how new ward managers translated the Blom-Cooper findings: 23 ward managers (WMs) were included (five were women and three appointed from outside the special hospitals to dilute its culture): one-third of the 18 male managers were also 'outsiders'. By open interviews, often going over a couple of days and audiotaped, structured questionnaire, shadowing them and attending their meetings, data were collected. By the end of 1992 there were at least 42 Ashworth working parties. A satirical note was circulated: 'if lonely hold a meeting . . . practical alternative to work'.

Managers new to Ashworth were sabotaged: nurses hid their mail and worked to rule, and the females had threatening mock attacks made on their wards in the dark. The power demarcation swung in favour of the patient, all complaints had to have detailed responses. One ward manager flippantly answered complaints 'that the radiator is talking to me' and a 'nurse served my potatoes with a sneer'. He was disciplined. Patients formed ward committees and Ashworth had a hospital patients' committee, supported by an external advocacy service. Demands came from some patients for same sex and others in their rooms.

An expensive consultancy firm and task force were drafted into the hospital, to assist the new WMs. After an initial honeymoon they became hostile towards the consultants. They discussed how they came out of the first meeting with them 'on cloud 9'; they were told how important they were. Expensive suits replaced casual wear; executive cases became the norm; they created their own forums, and money was allocated to them to construct their own modular ward management course. A forum meeting 7 May 1993 debated whether it should be a certificate or a diploma.

From my notes at the time, I find a list of sources of WM hostility about the expensive consultancy firm. External consultants did not support ward managers' political agenda of being incorporated into the higher management group (HMG), making hospital strategic decisions, after they fulfilled all their own targets. They reduced costs by appointing lower-grade nurses; reduced the overtime bill; themselves put in countless hours of unpaid overtime; developed alliances with other WMs for share costing; made unpleasant decisions in selecting new team leaders etc. The consultants responded by calling a meeting on 'group working' (25 January 1993) and to the managers' disgust played 'trivial' icebreaker exercises with matches!! The managers 'rebelled' and told the consultants, 'What is the common theme of WMs? Our relations with our seniors' (Richman and Mercer, 2000). When some WMs became candidates for disciplinary action, the co-existence with HMG ended. Disillusionment set in, with WMs now regarding their role as 'fall guys' for Ashworth's ills, now and future.

From the WMs' perspective, the consultants were discredited. They were viewed as hospital outsiders, not conversant with the forensic tradition, rarely visiting the wards to 'admire' the new regimes, thus lacking special hospital credibility – their alienability was a major handicap. Consultants were not interested in WMs' budget dilemmas: fundholding was a new concept. One manager said, 'I would like complete responsibility for my own ward. I haven't got that; with a budget of £250 000, most is spoken for'! When HMG unilaterally withdrew £1000 for each ward's budget they considered it theft/being mugged, especially after they had lengthy negotiations with patients on how to spend the money.

The forum meeting (4 June 1993) discussed how the 'flexible' budget element had still never been reconciled. If the HMG never gave a clear response they agreed to go 'outside', to the Special Hospital Strategic Group (SHSG), the government body. Also, doctors were not fundholders, but made patient arrangements with budget implications, e.g. 24 hours 'specialling' involved nine staff for one potential suicide (who told me he intended to bankrupt the ward!). Seventy-six per cent (16) WMs wanted doctors to be budget holders.

Consultants accepted uncritically all the findings of the Blom-Cooper Inquiry. Only two WMs accepted 'uncritically' the findings. Many of the complaints referred to the old Moss Side (South and East Ashworth) but not North (old Park Lane). The report made 'mistakes', which the inquiry would not later publish. For example, a named charge nurse from Newman, a ward for the elderly, was mistaken for someone else. She was a dedicated Christian and was easily cleared of misconduct. The consultants did not give support.

The consultants claimed credit for innovations by others. For example WMs were deficient in IT and quality assurance skills, and the consultants would not provide in-service training. WMs brought in their own expertises, for example. The consultants claimed credit for innovations such as this. Of the HMG's investment in consultants to initiate the 'new era', Machiavelli's words in *The Prince* are apt: 'A prince who is not himself wise cannot be wisely advised . . . good advice depends on the shrewdness of the prince who seeks it'!

A task force headed by a prestigious nurse, Malcolm Rae, was drafted in; each member headed a specific task. They were visible, especially on the wards. Their task was to bring in the 'culture change': 'the abandonment of the unhappy past' (Blom-Cooper *et al.*, vol. 1, p.253). One WM was totally in favour of the task force; the others negative. The task force set each WM 24 questions about their changes and then interviewed them, often for a couple of days. The WMs initially saw the task force as allies, hoping that their innovations would be sponsored. I was co-opted and used my accountant friends to produce financial projections etc for the WMs' intensive care unit, a facility for crisis intervention to stabilise patients. One argued that '11.1% of patients absorbed 41.7% of his ward's nursing input', which was seen to be unfair on the rest of the patients. Some of the WMs were co-opted onto the task force. That the task force's contract was not going to be renewed at the end of 6 months meant that they (like the external consultants) were not likely to be around when the changes they recommended were initiated.

The post Blom-Cooper period was also one of active, interprofessional disputes, for the system had been opened up. Rehabilitation changed its practitioners' name to 'therapist'; the psychologists staked claims to be the treatment leaders, subordinating doctors. My own survey of WMs (unpublished, March 1993) showed that 48% (11) rated patient care as considerably improved; 35% (8) argued 'moderate gains'; one manager said there were none. This improvement was not due to external inputs, ran the argument. The task force encouraged 24 hours' care to 'normalise' patients. This undermined the ward regimes. Patients stayed up all night playing videos and were too tired in the morning to go to workshops, part of their care plans. That the task force appropriated others' ideas was common. The task force adopted a WMs' admission scheme as a model for all wards to follow.

Post Blom-Cooper there was no corporate strategy for dealing collectively with its 90 recommendations; most were overlapping, especially on equal opportunities. The task force and external consultants appeared to be HMG committees. They did nothing to stop the wards being inundated with paper – protocols for this and that. By 1994 the WMs' morale was at a low ebb. Some were on long-term sickness others were looking for new jobs. 'If the paperwork is correct the organisation is functioning well', was the new logic.

My last days in Ashworth

The last research outing was in examining how nurses make care plans from medical records. This was a collective effort, with two Ashworth colleagues. It involved vignette research and I did the interviewing. Serendipity produced staff classifications of the 'evil' patient. This was the everyday language of PCTMs. I have heard psychiatrists say: 'the only way he is going to leave here is in a box'. Or nurses exclaim when confronted with a case vignette: 'he is evil, throw away the key'! Psychotic/schizophrenic patients were not labelled 'evil' because they did not 'own their heads'. But those, for example, whose offences were planned and committed over time, were (Richman *et al.*, 1999).

The research in the special hospital was terminated by a serious illness, involving 6 months of hospitalisation. Being disabled, walking with sticks, is not the ideal way of doing field work in Ashworth, especially in the post-Blom-Cooper period when, for the first time, I never felt safe on the wards – the frontier of control being one of changing sinuosity. Also, I did not feel like battling with the newly established ethics committee, with its party line on 'suitable research', as my colleagues discovered. Douglas (1972) refers to 'entrance barriers' as 'fronts'. The longer you linger by fronts, the more research intent is distorted.

In writing this retrospective account, this view of Oleson has resonated with me:

Invoking one's past is not the easiest of tasks: one anguishes over sins of omission and commission and recoils in embarrassment or guilt over images of the self in past fieldwork. Yet some unrepentant (or perhaps reborn) part of the field-worker surges to the fore in consciousness and anticipates the next ethnographic adventure.

(Oleson, 1990, p.227)

Ashworth taught me that there are times when you cannot always be cocooned in the research role: obeying 'methodological orders'. During probably my last field work in a category 'A' prison, focusing on palliative care, especially for the elderly prisoner, I had no regrets in crossing the line by criticising things. Then the governor 'advised' me to leave. That patients with severe depression should be 'banged up' for 22 hours a day at weekends was an anathema.

Concluding, by resurrecting primarily my earlier Ashworth ventures I have avoided producing a retrospective theoretical reading of my field data, supplementing it lavishly with the weaknesses or strengths of others. Instead I deployed what Althusser (Elliott, 1987) calls 'symptomatic reading'; what is at stake here is not completeness or consistency but the manner of the research seeing itself. My triangulation points for accounts are sometimes determined for me; some are my choice of 'critical junctures'. The ghosts of Ashworth will always haunt me.

References

Boynton J (1980) *Report of the Review of Rampton Hospital.* Cmnd 8073. London: HMSO.

Blom-Cooper L, Brown M, Dolan R and Murphy E (1992) *Report of the Committee of Inquiry into Complaints about Ashworth Hospital.* Cm 2028. London: HMSO.

Caldwell G and Naismith C (1989) Violent incidents on special care wards. *Medical Science and Law* **7**: 117–21.

Caudill W (1958) *The Psychiatric Hospital as a Small Society.* Harvard: Harvard University Press.

Dachelet CZ, Wemett MF, Garling EJ *et al.* (1981) The critical incident technique as applied to the evaluation of clinical practicum setting. *Journal of Nursing Education* **20**: 15–31.

Douglas D (1972) Managing fronts in observing deviance. In: Douglas JD (ed.) Research on Deviance. New York: Random House, pp. 73–95.

Elliott G (1987) *Althusser: the detour of theory.* London: Verso.

Evans-Pritchard EE (1937) *Witchcraft, Oracles and Magic among the Azande.* Oxford: Clarendon Press.

Goffman E (1968) *Asylums: essay on the social situation of mental patients and other inmates.* Harmondsworth: Penguin.

Gouldner AW (1954) *Wildcat Strike. A study in worker–management relations.* London: Harper Row.

Hammond PE (1964) *Sociologists at Work.* New York: Basic Books.

Henry J (1958) Space and power on a psychiatric unit. In: Jaco EG (ed.) *Patients, Physicians and Illness.* Illinois: Free Press, pp. 111–29.

Home Office (1991) *Prison Disturbances, April 1990: report of an inquiry by the Rt Hon Lord Justice Woolf (Parts 1 and 2) and His Honour Judge Stephen Tumin (Part 3).* Cmnd 1456. London: HMSO.

Hunter C (1988) *A Treatment Regime for Psychopaths.* Paper presented to the Conference on the Anti-Social Personality: research assessments and treatment programmes, 18 August 1988, at the Highland Inn, Midland, Ontario, Canada.

Lees GD, Richman J, Salaroo MA and Warden S (1987) Quality assurance: is it professional insurance? *Journal of Advanced Nursing* 12: 719–27.

Lofland LH (1989) On Fieldwork, Erving Goffman (transcribed and edited by Lyn H Lofland, with permission of Gillian Sankoff, Goffman's widow). *Journal of Contemporary Ethnography* **18**: 123–32.

Martin JP (1984) *Hospitals in Trouble*. Oxford: Basil Blackwell.

Mercer D and Richman J (2006) Scapegoat, spectacle and confessional: close encounters with sex offenders and other species of dangerous individuals. In: Mason T (ed.) *Forensic Psychiatry, Influences of Evil*. New Jersey: Humana Press, pp. 51–80.

Moos R and Hoots P (1968) The assessment of social atmospheres of psychiatric wards. *Journal of Abnormal Psychology* **73**: 595–604.

Olesen V (1990) Immersed, amorphous and episodic field work: theory and policy in three contrasting contexts. In: W. Burgess W (ed.) *Studies in Qualitative Methodology Vol. 2*. London: Jai Press, pp. 205–32.

Pollner M and Emerson RM (1983) The dynamics of inclusion and distance in fieldwork relations. In: Emerson RM (ed.) *Contemporary Field Research: a collection of readings*. Boston: Little John, pp. 25–41.

Richman J (1987) *Staff Attitudes of Park Lane and Cheadle Royal Hospitals Towards their Nursing Education Merger*. Unpublished NHS internal report.

Richman J (1989) *Psychiatric Ward Cultures Revisited: implications for treatment regimes*. Paper presented to the BSA Annual Conference, 12 September, Plymouth.

Richman J (1994) Male sociologist in a woman's world: aspects of a medical partnership. In: Burgess W (ed.) *Studies in Qualitative Methodology Vol. 4*. London: Jai Press, pp. 171–206.

Richman J (1997) The ceremonial and moral order of a ward for psychopaths. In: Mason T and Mercer D (eds) *Critical Perspectives in Forensic Care. Inside out*. Basingstoke: Macmillan, pp. 81–109.

Richman J and Mason T (1992) Quo vadis the special hospitals? In: Scott S, Williams G, Platt S and Thomas H (eds) *Private Risks and Public Dangers*. Aldershot: Avebury, pp. 150–67.

Richman J and Mercer D (2000) Rites of purification: the aftermath of the Ashworth Hospital Inquiry of 1992. *Journal of Forensic Psychiatry* **11**: 621–46.

Richman J and Mercer D (2001) Ward managers' attitudes towards external consultants in Ashworth, a special hospital, 1992–1994. *Health Services Management Research* **14**: 141–6.

Rosenhan DL (1973) On being sane in insane places. *Science* **179**: 250–8.

Stanton HA and Schwartz MS (1954) *The Mental Hospital: a study of institutional participation in psychiatric illness and treatment.* New York: Basic Books.

Thrasher J and Smith HL (1964) Interactional contexts of psychiatric patients: social roles and organisational implications. *Psychiatry* **27**: 389–98.

Van Maanen J (1988) *Tales of the Field: on writing ethnography*. Chicago: University of Chicago Press.

Wieder DL (1974) *Language and Social Reality: the case of telling the convict code*. The Hague: Mouton.

Chapter 4

Psychosocial interventions at Ashworth: an occupational delusion

Mick McKeown

Introduction

I worked at Ashworth between 1991 and 1995 as a nurse therapist in a centrally located rehabilitation unit. There were two of these rehabilitation centres, situated in the North and South sites of the hospital campus, reflecting the previous configuration of services in two separate hospitals (*see* Chapter 1). The South Rehabilitation Centre was one of the few aspects of Ashworth that attracted positive comments in the Blom-Cooper Inquiry: 'Dr Sines and Mr Thompson singled out the environment of the rehabilitation department for praise, a well designed oasis of purposeful activity in a desert of bleak wards' (Blom-Cooper *et al.*, 1992, p.146).

The centre operated somewhat along the lines of a 'day hospital' within the hospital, with patients travelling from the wards to attend for specific groups or one-to-one psychotherapies. It was managed and staffed by a small team of nurses, who worked alongside other colleagues to plan and deliver interventions, often co-working in pairs to facilitate groups. There was a strong emphasis upon behavioural and cognitive-behavioural approaches informed by the work of Robert Ross and colleagues (Ross and Gendreau, 1980; Ross and Fabiano, 1985) in the Canadian correctional system and the developing UK evidence base for 'what works' in offender therapy (McGuire, 1995). Indeed, the clinical psychologist James McGuire, one of the leading lights in this field, worked in Ashworth at the time and made a significant contribution to the work of the centre. Following the Blom-Cooper Inquiry, there was an impetus to develop an additional rehabilitation centre located in the North site of the hospital, and it was here that I was recruited to work.

Another member of the new team staffing the North centre was Ged McCann, who already had an extensive career within Ashworth and brought with him an interest in psychosocial approaches and a commitment to better meeting the needs of relatives of people detained in secure hospitals. Building upon previous work in the hospital, Ged inspired and instigated further efforts that were eventually to lead to the proposals which are the subject of this chapter.

The attempt at innovation

At the time we are concerned with here, there was a growing bandwagon in UK mental health care to adopt psychosocial approaches into routine services. This was so much the case that psychosocial interventions (PSI) have been referred to as a 'new wave' of psychological treatment. Though these efforts were largely focused upon mainstream community services, subsequently there has been a similar push to adopt psychosocial interventions into inpatient settings. In the mid-1990s there was sufficient momentum of research findings to help secure a grant from the Sir Jules Thorn Charitable Trust to establish the first systematic training courses in psychosocial interventions.

This 'Thorn' course was started in two centres, at the University of Manchester and the Institute of Psychiatry, London, itself grounded in earlier training initiatives led, respectively, by Nick Tarrier at Manchester and Julien Leff in London (Leff, 2000). The Thorn model of delivering psychosocial training has since spread out to be taught at a number of places across the country, in a cascade model of dissemination (O'Carroll *et al.*, 2004). This in some way endorses the original 'premise that some of the trainees coming to the London and Manchester centres would be of sufficient calibre to establish satellite training centres in their home bases' (Leff, 2000, p.250).

The original Thorn courses recruited practitioners in pairs from their host teams, on the assumption that they would be better able to support each other in post-training implementation of new working practices, and might be better placed to establish satellite training centres (Leff, 2000). Ged McCann and I managed to secure places in the second cohort of trainees at the Manchester Thorn course in 1994, despite the criteria being for community staff only at this time. We were able to do this because we had already demonstrated an interest in developing psychosocial approaches in the high-security setting, and had previously initiated project work and associated inquiry in this regard. Building upon Ged's earlier work looking at the needs of families with relatives detained in places like Ashworth, this work gathered pace during and after our time on the course, culminating in us inviting senior staff associated with the Manchester Thorn course to assist us in training and developing a small team at Ashworth. This initiative helped us to further develop ideas about adapting the psychosocial model to practice within a secure setting, and led to us undertake a number of small-scale but interesting research studies.

Organic training

The organic approach to training and development builds upon our earliest reflections upon the challenges presented by attempting to use training to usher in practice change, especially within a secure setting. Various authors have remarked upon the relative gap between training outcomes for individual practitioners (very good) and service level outcomes regarding the uptake of new ideas into routine practice (typically very poor). For instance, commentators have remarked upon the fact that graduates of training courses face an unfair burden in attempting to enact practice change, services are not best organised to facilitate such a contribution, and evaluation of the impact of training is typically inadequate (Fadden, 1997; Gournay and Sandford, 1998; McKeown *et al.*, 2002). In the US, Corrigan and McCracken (1995) identified a number of fundamental barriers to the implementation of improved ways of working in inpatient environments. These include:

- bureaucratic constraints
- accessibility of effective treatments
- insufficient numbers of well-trained personnel.

Our organic model of training aims to tackle these barriers to practice change by drawing upon various theories of interactive learning and development that employ 'action' principles, including the interactive staff-training approach advocated by Corrigan and colleagues (Corrigan and McCracken, 1995; Corrigan *et al.*, 1997) and models of appreciative inquiry (*see* Cooperrider and Srivastva 1987). Importantly, these approaches are designed to avoid a number of obvious pitfalls with more traditional models of training. Such training can appear to proceed solely from an implicit or explicit criticism of the status quo, immediately setting up staff resistance to contemplation of change. Similarly, staff can feel that blueprints or manifestos for change are pre-ordained, leaving little opportunity to develop a stake in or ownership of any resulting proposals.

These points are important in a context of secure care, where often new ideas can be challenged as to their transferability from other settings where they may have been originally conceived (as with PSI) and/or suitability for a forensic client group. There may also be something of a siege mentality amongst staff who are wary of repeated exhortations that practice must change without any sense that concerted effort has gone into understanding the complexities and practicalities of delivering appropriate care in this setting. A dimension of this latter point might also translate into scepticism, or even outright hostility, towards trainers who appear to be beamed in from outside without having the assumed credibility of shared knowledge of the practice environment, i.e. they face the accusatory declamation: 'If you haven't worked here, or in a place like this, what can you contribute?'.

The proposal

Our proposals for the implementation of psychosocial approaches at Ashworth had a number of interlinked strands. These included:

- a forensic 'Thorn' Diploma and other supportive training to be delivered on-site at Ashworth. This would utilise the well-appointed staff education centre and also include team training delivered on wards
- adoption of psychosocial approaches into routine practice across the two mental illness directorates. This would involve:
  - a system of multidisciplinary case management
  - routine use of a range of appropriate assessment tools
  - delivery of a range of psychological interventions for the amelioration of symptoms of psychosis
  - meeting the needs of relatives and their appropriate involvement in care of their family member

- a programme of research to evaluate and explore:
    - the effectiveness of the training course
    - the effectiveness of psychosocial interventions in the high-security setting
    - psychotic experiences and their link with offending
    - psychosocial stress on wards, including staff–patient encounters.

We presented a paper at a special seminar of the Forensic Psychiatric Nurses Association (FPNA), held at Ashworth on 3 March 1995, a version of which was eventually published in *Psychiatric Care*, the house journal of the FPNA at the time (McCann and McKeown, 1995). This paper was written and presented at the conference in the middle of our efforts to secure support for the project, and reflects our optimism and enthusiasm for its potential. Ironically, by the time of its publication in the journal, efforts to secure support for the proposals had irretrievably foundered and both Ged and myself had left the employment of Ashworth. The paper that was eventually published indicated our affiliations in new jobs elsewhere.

In this paper we described the national 'Thorn' initiative and detailed how, in our view, this could be translated into a secure setting. We outlined what we felt to be a persuasive rationale for this which, amongst other things, suggested that the high-security setting needed the introduction of psychosocial approaches, not least because of the high proportion (around 70%) of patients diagnosed with psychosis. This reasoning included the implications for practice contained in various extant reports and reviews of forensic care and wider mental health services, including the (at the time) recently published Butterworth Report (Mental Health Nursing Review Team, 1994) into the future of mental health nursing, and the Reed Review (1994) of secure care, recommending a refocusing of nursing time towards the care of people with the most severe mental health problems. We also offered a critique of current levels of service provision for this client group in Ashworth, and detailed a number of expected benefits that might be assumed to flow from reorganising and improving these services.

We argued that:

- the introduction of psychosocial approaches and associated systems of case management would bring the high-security setting in line with developments elsewhere in the NHS, promoting the notion of seamless services across different care agencies. Effective systems of case management would also offer new and possibly more interesting roles for staff, particularly ward-based nurses. Implementation ought also to offer individual patients a better sense of their progress through a care and treatment system, possibly offering an implicit incentive for more active engagement
- best practice in multidisciplinary working and case management would be greatly assisted by the necessary adoption of a unitary conceptual framework or model across all relevant wards. The status quo involved a number of wards operating different nursing models of care, many of which were opaque or meaningless to other disciplines and quite often, arguably, irrelevant to the client group or setting
- despite the evidence base for psychosocial approaches being mainly located in community practice, large numbers of people with severe and enduring mental health problems remained in some form of institutional care, and that these concentrations were exaggerated in the forensic system

- at Ashworth there was an almost complete absence of psychosocial approaches and many individuals continued to experience positive symptoms of psychosis despite widespread use of neuroleptic drugs (often in large doses)
- relatively long periods of admission ought to support the establishment of strong therapeutic alliances, opportunities for continuity of care, and the application of programmatic PSI case work
- there was a lack of attention to the needs of families, and family members were not routinely involved in the care of their relatives. A consequence of this was that many relatives and patients had low expectations of services and poor opinions of the hospital and its care
- external research and findings from our own studies undertaken within Ashworth provided a starting point for contemplation of improved services
- nurses could be easily located as key figures in the social network of detained individuals. Yet, despite being ideally placed, they were often poorly equipped to address issues of stress mediation at ward level
- for patients at Ashworth at the time, assessment and evaluation of progress was piecemeal, *ad hoc*, and inconsistent and, despite availability for the role, nurses were not routinely undertaking formal assessments
- many nurses wished to address these issues and were often supported to take on further training. The impact of current training was difficult to quantify, and in any event the choice of training courses was typically unplanned and unsystematic, being led by practitioner demand rather than a well-thought out strategy. For example, nurses would undertake the sort of counselling course that did not have demonstrable value in meeting the needs of this client group
- prevailing recruitment problems for clinical psychologists were limiting the availability of psychological therapies at Ashworth. The introduction of a planned and systematic psychosocial service could both promote and extend the sort of collegiate multidisciplinary working evident in the rehabilitation centres, and also possibly render the hospital more attractive to potential recruits.

We went on to outline what a Thorn initiative would actually involve in a forensic setting. We envisaged an emphasis upon a stress-vulnerability model of care, with implications at ward level for providing interventions focused upon stress in the ward environment. This would involve the care team working towards identification of significant psychosocial stress factors for individuals, and working alongside them to develop coping strategies to monitor and deal with stress. Staff would also have to consider their own role in mediating stress that might arise in their interactions with patients, leading to contemplation of expressed emotion in staff–patient encounters (more about this below). The aim would be to promote distinctly low-expressed emotion ward atmospheres grounded in staff's effective use of simple communication skills.

We envisaged the wholesale adoption of a thorough case management approach, including the use of a range of accurate and reliable assessment tools and proper attention to principles of effective engagement and therapeutic relationship building. Staff training in this regard would focus upon skills relevant to assessing:

- mental health needs
- social functioning

- specific behavioural problems
- effects of medication
- positive and negative symptoms (and the impact on people's lives)
- needs of relatives.

At this time, there was not a well-established tradition of nurses being heavily involved in the use of systematic assessments of individual functioning and experience of symptoms. The Thorn initiative nationally had made the case for nurses extending their role to become more accomplished and consistent in the reliable use of such assessment tools, and hence then be better placed to accurately identify problems, needs, and strengths and more fully engage in multidisciplinary case discussions and care planning. This argument could be extended in our view to specific issues pertinent to forensic settings regarding the need for more thorough assessment of risk, particularly dangerousness and the risk of re-offending. Possibly the best case for implementation of a forensic Thorn initiative was the opportunity to develop new knowledge in the psychological management of symptoms, particularly in a context where large numbers of individuals were deemed to be resistant to other forms of therapy. The growing evidence for the effectiveness of cognitive-behavioural approaches to the management of positive psychotic symptoms suggested the value of adopting interventions aimed at, for example:

- psycho-education as a basis for self-management
- self-monitoring of symptoms
- assessment of antecedents and behaviours associated with symptoms
- development of specific coping strategies
- focusing techniques for auditory hallucinations
- belief modification strategies with delusions
- cognitive approaches for thought disorder.

We argued that if the implementation of such interventions was also properly researched, we might be able to demonstrate both that interventions developed elsewhere had utility in forensic settings, and that new knowledge might emerge that illuminated possible linkages between the experience of psychosis and the commission of particular offences.

It was our contention at the time that the successful implementation of psychosocial interventions at Ashworth required a plan for large-scale and systematic transformational change. In other words, it was no use tinkering about the edges or impeding possible benefits by introducing piecemeal changes. The emphasis accorded to establishing key principles in case management would hopefully support a co-ordinated and consistent application of the proposed initiatives across the relevant directorates of the hospital. We envisaged and planned for a progressive development of the whole service, with roughly 12 staff recruited to undertake the full diploma each year, while others would be trained to support the ethos and practice of psychosocial interventions and how to use various assessment tools in a process of continuing education. Over time, the numbers of individuals receiving psychosocial interventions would increase.

We were interested in persuading staff, clinicians and managers at the hospital of a number of anticipated benefits we felt would follow from establishing such a forensic 'Thorn' initiative. Training nursing staff to undertake systematic assessments and deliver psychosocial interventions would hugely increase the volume of therapy available to patients, especially at ward level. The acknowledged relative lack of clinical psychology input could be offset by the contribution of nurses, and the introduction of a service grounded in psychological models could concomitantly assist in recruitment. Training and supervision could directly address psychosocial stress on wards, enabling staff to ameliorate stress in the ward environment, with possible improvements in morale for both patients and staff.

This raised the potential for wards to be recast as centres of therapy, rather than merely residences or places of containment, with therapeutic endeavours typically being enacted elsewhere or being the sole province of practitioners based away from the wards. Any increase in psychosocial therapies would prove to be an important adjunct to medical intervention. Shifting the basis of assessment onto a more rational and systematic basis would enhance the information brought forward within care teams in discussion of progress and future care planning. If nurses, in particular, were able to demonstrate proficiency in these and other skills, then there might also be opportunities for more respectful and democratic relationships within care teams, leading to better and more effective multidisciplinary team working.

The psychosocial approach also offers the potential for democratising staff–patient relationships, ushering in new models of therapeutic alliance. Individuals and their families could be supported to be much more informed and involved in their own care. We argued at the time that this could have offered Ashworth a leading role in developing new ways of working in forensic care that improved partnerships in treatment and care delivery.

Around this time we were also involved in setting up the first conference of its kind in a high-security setting that focused upon user involvement and empowerment in forensic care, and facilitated participation of patients, relatives and staff in the proceedings (Chapman and McKeown, 1994). Contemporaneously, the emerging 'hearing voices' movement was becoming increasingly influential in mainstream mental health services (Romme *et al.*, 1992), offering new insights for practitioners concerned with notions of therapeutic alliance. Reflecting on this now, at a time when NHS policy rhetoric is replete with notions of partnership, participation and user involvement (and secure care settings are typically cast as lagging behind), it is acutely disappointing that we were not afforded the chance to develop these particular ideas further.

Other organisational benefits could be imagined. With the contemporary development of particular commissioning arrangements meaning that hospitals like Ashworth had to be more explicit about the specifics of treatment packages to justify costs and outcomes, the idea of a systematic approach to care and treatment for the majority client group ought to have been singularly attractive to hospital managers. There would also probably have been some significant positive public relations spin-offs for a hospital beleaguered by bad press at this time.

Institutional resistance

From the outset, we were aware that actually achieving the support to implement our ideas would not necessarily be a smooth ride. We made some progress in persuading staff, senior clinicians and managers of the merits of the proposals. We had drawn up a fully costed business plan and had begun to attend various team, executive and directorate meetings to assist in making the case and answer challenging questions. We had also secured the provisional support of colleagues at the University of Manchester that the Thorn initiative would be happy to seek validation of a Forensic Thorn Diploma as a satellite course within a cascade model of dissemination.

At this time we remained confident of the value of the plan and were reasonably optimistic that the proposals would be supported sufficiently to be allowed to make a start with implementation. A number of significant people within the various hierarchies had expressed support for the plans, including senior clinicians and managers. There were, however, some equally senior individuals who were not backing us, and it turns out, some of these were attacking the plan behind the scenes (i.e. not in formal meetings to which we were invited).

At this time, while we were actively pursuing support for the proposals, the experience was such that we wrote:

> Attempting to get this proposal off the ground has involved selling the idea to management and other practitioners. As in any large organisation there has been some institutional inertia to change, manifesting in some instances as resistance to the scheme. There has also been evident a degree of ignorance about the approach and the supporting research. This can impact upon purchasing decisions if the individuals charged with purchasing responsibility do not have a true picture of an initiative's worth. Such problems are exacerbated when, as is often the case, management becomes divorced from clinical practice, especially from external developments. An historical tendency towards rigid interdisciplinary demarcation at Ashworth (Blom-Cooper *et al.*, 1992) could also impinge upon the eventual success of the scheme by undermining effective multidisciplinary working.
> (McCann and McKeown, 1995, p.136)

So there was a mixture of support and resistance; in a place like Ashworth, or any large concern for that matter, it would be typically so. We would have been comfortable with this if the only issues at stake were the actual merits or otherwise of the proposals. Subsequent events suggesting that this was not wholly the case exacerbated the eventual disappointment and frustration of not managing to secure sufficient support to establish the project.

Ged and I wrote the business case for the proposal, and costings were provided by a management accountant working for the hospital on the direction of the senior nursing manager at Ashworth at the time. Given the recently introduced clinical directorates at Ashworth (mental illness (×2), personality disorder, women's services and rehabilitation), a number of noteworthy complications arose for our plans. Firstly, the act of securing approval for the proposals became more complex, in that rather than having to persuade a single management board and a single medical executive team, we had to do all of this *and* secure the approval of *both* the mental illness directorates' management teams *and* senior clinicians.

Interestingly, we were told that the project could not proceed in just one of the mental illness directorates: if one supported and one did not (which, indeed, was eventually the case), the proposal would fall. The stakes were all or nothing: unless there was unanimous support there was to be no project. This stance was eventually rationalised on the basis that the evidence base for the proposals was not fully demonstrated within high-security settings, so the senior personnel had to be wholly persuaded of the merits of transferability, with evaluation running parallel, and that any doubts would fatally undermine the project. So we were faced with a chicken and egg scenario: no specific research demonstrating effectiveness is located in a forensic setting, hence you cannot start to implement services 'without an evidence base'; but, unless a start is made there would be no opportunity to develop a peculiarly forensic evidence base.

The fact that we had already undertaken some, albeit small-scale, studies was dismissed, as was the potentially equally persuasive logic of contesting the absolute claim to 'special' status afforded to the forensic client. One could present an argument that the experience of psychosis, and hence its psychosocial treatment, had sufficient commonalities across treatment settings to at least justify an attempt to demonstrate effectiveness. Cynically, it could also be argued that as long as the proposed psychosocial initiative was not likely to do any harm, then it was worth a try on the basis of the previously remarked upon relative dearth of therapeutic activity across the wards of an institution that was in this sense undeserving of the name 'hospital'. In the end it was this rather tautological logic of unproven forensic effectiveness that defeated us; but it is highly debatable whether such a test was either justified or even the real rationale for failing to support the initiative.

The other complication arising from the restructuring of the hospital into directorates that arose at this time really ought to have assisted the bid. The rehabilitation centres did not fit easily into the new structures, especially given the need for each directorate to develop its own 'identity' and take charge of its own therapeutic direction. The idea of a central resource that patients travelled to from their wards but was managed elsewhere was not to be easily accommodated in a new culture of distinct directorates. One of the possible solutions for this managerial problem that was floated around this time was that the rehabilitation centres would be disbanded and the staff would be dispersed to new roles within different directorates.

Given that our jobs as they stood were possibly effectively being made redundant, our proposals would have redirected Ged's and my posts to the new 'Thorn' initiative as an alternative to dropping into a (as yet undefined) post in one of the directorates. In our view, this rendered the actual costs of funding our proposals really quite affordable. The major costs would be our salaries, and these could be redirected from essentially redundant roles. The additional revenue costs in the project were to be no more than around £5000 annually.

Reflecting upon our contemporaneous feeling that some of the resistance to the project was borne out of ignorance (that some people did not appreciate the true value of the proposals) brings us back into contemplation of the insularity of large, closed institutions like Ashworth. I noted earlier that in the early to mid-1990s there was a growing bandwagon coalescing around psychosocial interventions. Arguably, a case could be made that even the wider NHS had actually been slow on the uptake in recognising the merit of previous research in this regard.

But, more recently, you would be hard pressed to find a set of interventions more fashionable in the history of UK mental health care than the vogue for cognitive-behavioural therapy (CBT). Much of the enthusiasm for these psycho-social approaches was already widespread in the NHS at the time of our proposals, yet, despite this, we found that numerous practitioners were simply unaware of either the evidence base or the associated policy noise.

Some others were aware of these matters but had a distorted view of the research, feeling that it could not be applied to the most treatment-resistant indi-viduals, i.e. those detained at Ashworth. A variant on this critical perspective was the arguably unimaginative stance – those people who could see the value of psychosocial interventions elsewhere but who simply could not contemplate the possible adaptations that would render them useful in a place like Ashworth. An example of this would be to see the value of family interventions, but to deny that these would be of any use in a high-security hospital because of the limited contact time with relatives.

Hence, two possible avenues for the development of a forensic psychosocial interventions initiative were closed down for lack of creative imagination. First, one could consider the particular needs of relatives in the special circumstances of high-security care, and the contribution that they could make to, for example, assisting care teams to better understand the offending behaviour that led to admission in the first place, or the value of involving relatives in pre-discharge planning if they are likely to have a continuing role in social support. Second, the whole notion of the psychosocial environment of the hospital and the contribu-tion of staff–patient relationships to ward atmosphere and psychosocial stress is neglected.

So one interpretation of the failure to persuade a critical mass of decision makers of the value of our proposals is the possibility, remarked upon often else-where, that the nature of the institution was to be relatively closed off from new ideas (however popular beyond the walls). Similarly, if novel ideas could pene-trate the closed institution, there would be suspicion and scepticism that models of care developed in non-forensic settings could be of any use in the 'special' environment within the walls. The recognition, in a broad sense, that such atti-tudes prevailed in total institutions such as Ashworth is implicitly acknowledged in the recent moves to limit their independence and incorporate their operational management into mainstream NHS trusts.

The fact that Ashworth experienced not one but two public inquiries that book-ended the period we are talking about, suggests that there were systemic problems with the workforce and the judgement of various senior managers and clinicians. A number of the people we engaged with in our struggle to initiate our project were explicitly criticised in the later Fallon Inquiry (Fallon *et al.*, 1999), and at least one of the individuals who was to prove a major stumbling block for us eventually lost his job as a direct result of the exposure of his professional limi-tations in the Fallon Inquiry report. This senior clinical psychologist in one of the mental illness directorates spoke favourably about our project to my face and broadly speaking backed it in the context of public meetings, yet circulated an email that was extremely critical of the proposals and probably contributed to the subsequent failure of that directorate to support the project.

Though a leaked a copy of this email eventually emerged, we were not included in the original circulation so were effectively denied the opportunity to challenge its contents (which, amongst other things, pointedly questioned the capability of nurses in Ashworth to take on the skills and roles outlined in the proposal). This approach to communication seems particularly cowardly, and is in my view probably best described as an act of sabotage. My appreciation of life at Ashworth is such that I do not believe that this was a unique scenario, and in many ways it resonates with some of the ways in which patients experienced the system, for example in terms of their exclusion from open discussions around their care and progress in the system. It did not, however, necessarily require gross unprofessionalism to derail our plans. Perhaps we also suffered from standard low-level, mundane mismanagement and the occasional petty jealousies and personal protectionisms that were also a general feature of institutional life at Ashworth.

When we highlighted in our paper the idea that, in our opinion, management at Ashworth becomes divorced from clinical practice, especially from external developments, we were clearly aware at the time of the stifling effect of internal ignorance of ideas that were gaining massive currency outside of the institution. We were also remarking on an often-observed fact that, even in more enlightened circumstances, managers' priorities can lead them away from the cutting edge of clinical innovation. Individuals who have a range of pressures and competing objectives can often become distant from anything other than their day-to-day management role.

A classic management tactic employed at Ashworth in my time there, and clearly not unique to these institutions, was 'leave it with me!'. Only, of course, there was seldom any return to the topic, such that the impression given was that ideas could be flagged up but they would never be acted on. Of course, if such practices are also in a context of managers divorced from clinical reality, then there is a double whammy of frustration. My personal view is that some of my managerial colleagues at Ashworth at this time were not so much divorced from the reality of clinical practice (especially outside of a secure environment). Instead they might be best described as never having been married to this reality in the first place.

Too much of my experience at Ashworth leads me to conclude that nothing much was planned or thought out in advance. If it was, these plans were not transparent or shared with the workforce. Hence, even if it were not absolutely the case, the hospital management gave the appearance of aimlessness, or reactive, knee-jerk responses to particular events and circumstances.

What was missing was any sense of concerted inspirational leadership, cognisant of the detailed complexity of the environment and circumstances and willing to engage with it. Instead, there was every appearance of seeming to be afraid of the enormity of such a challenge. There seemed to be a complete absence of any well-articulated vision for clinical progress, and hence the idea of proactive management was relegated to the platitudes of glossy brochures (which Ashworth was rather good at) but seldom made an appearance in the real world of therapeutic nihilism, biomedical monoculture, and the desertification of care practices across wards noted by Blom-Cooper.

That this could occur at a time when the special hospitals seemed to be very much better off in terms of spending and resources than their impoverished mainstream NHS counterparts, renders one's reflections bleaker still. The seeming absence of planning and vision is quite obviously evident in the (lack of) staff training strategy. As I have previously pointed out, the hospital had (and still has) an incredibly well-resourced staff training centre with an extensive library resource. Arguably, this centre was one of the best parts of the hospital in my time there, and some notably able tutors and managers of education led some interesting developments in creating forensic training courses accredited with partner universities.

Many staff, Ged and myself included, were generously supported to undertake a range of courses, hosted in-house or at a range of universities. It is my opinion, however, that almost all of this learning was completely led by individual staff interests, and was never linked to any managerial plan for workforce development or enhancements to clinical practice. So staff would learn new knowledge and skills, but they would return to their corner of the workplace with no supported plan or strategy to implement changes to working practices. There was no overarching master-plan about how all of the individual learning opportunities for staff would link up in practical terms on the ground.

Another problem facing individuals concerned with practice innovation in a place like Ashworth was the reluctance of elements in the institution to engage with any internally generated critique. This was especially evident in a timidity about the possibility that any of this critique might be aired or articulated in ways that might extrude into the world outside the walls. There was a definite sense that 'news management' was one of the priorities of Ashworth management. One might hazard a guess that it was the top priority of a succession of chief executives, and the ministers they were accountable to. A cynical observation might be that the various chief executives who lost their jobs did so as much for their failure to contain the news, as for the actual nature of the malpractice uncovered.

A number of commentators have pointed out the symbolic role of high-security hospitals in containing levels of public anxiety associated with serious offending behaviour (*see* McKeown and Stowell-Smith 2006). It can be argued that public anxiety is minimised when no stories emerge from within the walls of secure care: when these institutions are silent, the public is happiest. The patients are contained in conditions of high security, segregated away from wider society, and the psychiatric professionals offer the comforting illusion that they are knowledgeably and assuredly in charge of the management and safe containment (and possible discharge) of these dangerous individuals.

The emergence of critical accounts from the inside to the outside threatens this accommodation of public fears, and a mini-industry of news management is required.

In my time at Ashworth there was an active public relations department that fulfilled this role. Anecdotally, I can recall a senior academic researcher bemoaning that more money was spent on this news manipulation activity than was allocated to internally funded research projects and associated support. I can just about see the justification for all of this as a counter measure to the sort of sensationalist and intrusive tabloid stories that quite regularly emerge from institutions like Ashworth. These would usually be initiated by a disgruntled member of staff, typically vexed by a perception that security measures were being overly liberalised or that prevailing conditions were too 'cushy' for the incarcerated clientele and, more often than not, could probably be attributed to the malign influence of right wing elements in the POA.

However, these real-enough provocative elements in the POA were not the whole story. The news management machinery was also wheeled out in an attempt to influence or constrain academic activity and therapeutic innovation in the hospital. Hence, it was a requirement at the time to submit manuscript copies of journal articles for external publication for review by the public relations department. Invariably, this would result in dialogue aimed at toning down any critique and/or suggestions to include other material that might show the hospital in a better light.

Given that a number of our papers were concerned with studies into the experiences of relatives, and that many of these people had been less than happy in their relationships with the institution and the wider criminal justice system, if we were to report our research with integrity these narratives could not be altered. Yet, this is exactly what we were asked to do. We declined to alter anything and successfully resisted any editorial changes. In any event, our output was not in our view overly critical and could equally be read as a positive example of good practice that organically belonged to Ashworth.

Management or mismanagement was not our only stumbling block. Perhaps more importantly was the issue of rigid interdisciplinary demarcation, and in particular the exercise of medical executive power. At this point I would like to reiterate that in my experience of working at Ashworth I probably had close working relationships with some of the very best nurses, social workers, clinical psychologists and psychiatrists I have ever had the privilege of working with. It is probably also fair to say that, having worked elsewhere in NHS mental health services, many of the shortcomings of places like Ashworth are also evident elsewhere, albeit to a lesser degree. However, it is also true that I came across some colleagues at Ashworth who would have struggled to find employment in any even marginally better-managed or progressive environment. A longstanding tradition of promotion through the ranks had probably contributed to a number of senior managers holding posts for which they were eminently unqualified. I had the misfortune of some of these individuals figuring in the trees of line management relating to my post.

Similarly, problems in recruitment of psychiatrists, coupled with the pre-eminence of this role within the legal framework, offered the medical executive an almost unassailably privileged position within the Ashworth hierarchy. Unfortunately, one or two notable exceptions notwithstanding, the prevailing clinical philosophy of most of Ashworth's psychiatrists at the time was singularly wedded to a very narrow biomedical model. From my experience of attempting to develop research projects in Ashworth I was left with the view that medical executive power was often exercised to stifle initiatives that were not medically inspired and controlled.

On at least one occasion, an Ashworth psychiatrist who had argued against a research proposal of mine spoke to me about his reasons. He stated that he was really not to blame, but felt that he had to support the line of a more senior psychiatrist colleague who felt that the study (bizarrely in my view) was an attempt to usher in medical audit by the back door! This was for a study building upon an earlier survey (McKeown and Liebling, 1995), which would compare case records of individuals' history of illicit drug use with reports of the same in structured interviews. I felt at the time that this was a somewhat paranoid interpretation of the study's aims. At the risk of sounding paranoid myself, one could say that the failure to have this particular project approved was a consequence of some sort of conspiracy, at least as it was told to me! Unfortunately, whatever was actually going on, this is another example of having to face objections that are not explicitly voiced in the appropriate forum, closing off any opportunity for a reasoned debate.

Still a good idea?

Since the mid-1990s, a number of published papers have added to the literature supporting the introduction of psychosocial approaches to inpatient environments generally, wider secure care settings, and high-security hospitals specifically. A number of reviews have continued to make the case for the widespread adoption of psychosocial interventions, including within inpatient environments.

Recent studies link these interventions to the notion of recovery (Kuipers, 1996; Huxley *et al.*, 2000; Bustillo *et al.*, 2001; McCann, 2001). Thompson (2000) reviewed the care and treatment of those with a diagnosis of schizophrenia in conditions of high security, and included a section on psychosocial interventions. Walker (2004), based at Carstairs High Security Hospital in Scotland, surveyed the use of psychosocial interventions in the hospital, and reported upon a number of relevant research studies recently completed or in progress.

Carstairs is reported as attempting to address the systematic introduction of psychosocial approaches from around 2000 onwards. Walker describes the identification of staff skill deficits (largely around the use of CBT) and calls for more systematic training and linking training to staff supervision. She also remarks upon the institution's acceptance of the need for investment of resources in PSI and the largely positive attitude of staff towards these changes.

Isherwood *et al.* (2006) call for service developments and staff training to implement psychosocial approaches to the management of psychosis in medium-security services for men with learning disabilities. Somewhat ironically, the need for systematic approaches to staff training was taken up in the second Ashworth Public Inquiry with Professor Kevin Gournay, who called in the Fallon Report for 'the implementation of a training package similar to the Thorn Programme to underpin working with this group of [personality disordered] patients' (Fallon *et al.*, 1999).

The idea of high expressed emotion in staff–patient encounters continues to receive attention in a variety of settings, and a number of evaluations of relevant staff training programmes have been undertaken. In a review of psychosocial interventions published in 1996, Liz Kuipers argued that interventions to address staff–patient expressed emotion ought to be considered for inpatient settings, and that insufficient research had considered the relationship between this and aspects of the therapeutic alliance (Kuipers 1996).

Other researchers in the Netherlands have studied expressed emotion in staff–patient relationships from both the staff and patient perspectives, noting again the high levels of expressed emotion in some staff–patient relationships (Van Humbeeck *et al.*, 2001). In another Dutch study, Finnema and colleagues (1996) studied staff expressed emotion on long-stay wards, and found measurable benefits for patients as a consequence of a staff training programme. A study of nursing staff in Swedish forensic units found that nurses typically employed confronting interventions, and this is discussed in the light of the expressed emotion research, suggesting this might contribute to worsening of psychotic symptoms (Rask and Levander, 2001).

Willets and Leff (1997) found that a relatively brief training intervention for staff in community care facilities helped to promote better staff knowledge, use of resources and change-management strategies, but failed to make an impact upon staff expressed emotion, suggesting the need for more intensive and practice-based training. Whittaker and Stickley (2003) make some interesting observations in a descriptive piece about a mental health unit operating psycho-social approaches. They discuss in detail aspects of therapeutic relationships in a context of expressed emotion, offering insights into the care of individuals seen as 'difficult' or 'non-enaging' before recommending an interactional solution that feeds into supportive systems of staff supervision.

Ewers and colleagues (2002) conducted a training initiative in psychosocial interventions for staff working on a medium-security unit and found that staff became more positive in their attitudes towards patients and were less likely to experience negative aspects of stress in their caring role. Forster and colleagues (2003) have developed and validated a user-focused measure of staff expressed emotion as perceived by patients, which is offered as a useful tool for research or the audit of quality of care in inpatient environments.

Estelle Moore, who initiated the study of staff-expressed emotion in the UK with her groundbreaking PhD study, went on to work in Broadmoor High Secure Hospital, and together with other colleagues published a study of expressed emotion in relationships between staff and patients in this setting (Moore *et al.*, 2002). The main finding of this study is supportive of a link between staff-expressed emotion and patient outcomes in a forensic environment, and the authors call for better systems of staff supervision and attention to 'core charac-teristics of optimal relationships . . . even for those whose problems present the most enduring challenges' (Moore *et al.*, 2002, p.215). Taylor and Jones (2006) argue that processes of clinical governance in secure care services should include attention to confidential assessments of staff variables such as expressed emotion.

Working with families in secure settings is less extensively covered, and some commentators continue to stress the challenges faced, including limitations on time because of geographical dislocation from families (Thomson, 2000). Evans (2000) reports from a Welsh medium-security setting that relatives who are involved in structured interventions appreciate the opportunity for involvement and see it as valuable. MacInnes (2000) provides a rationale for family work in a forensic setting, presenting a case study and description of best practice in such family interventions. Geelan and Nickford (1999) surveyed all medium-security units in England and Wales and found limited use of family therapy. They con-clude that there is a strong need for relevant staff training, and that psychosocial family interventions ought to be readily translatable into the routine practice of most multidisciplinary forensic teams. An Australian paper describes the develop-ment of a family support project through the establishment of a nursing practice development unit in a secure care context (Jubb and Shanley, 2002). The authors define their initiative by its departure from a narrow medical model.

A number of researchers over a significant amount of time have explored the association of particular aspects of psychotic experiences with risk of violence and dangerousness (*see* Wessley *et al.*, 1993; Link and Steuve, 1994, 1998; Swanson *et al.*, 1996; Steadman *et al.*, 1998; Taylor *et al.*, 1998). Cognitive-behavioural therapies for psychotic symptoms have been demonstrated to be effective in mainstream populations (Tarrier *et al.*,1998) and have been latterly taken up in forensic practice. This includes interventions for individuals with auditory hallucinations (Bentall and Haddock 2000) and paranoid delusions (Ewers *et al.*, 2000).

Walker's (2004) account of psychosocial interventions in Carstairs emphasises CBT as a major element of developmental aspirations, but limited in practice by a shortage of appropriately trained staff. The Carstairs initiative has developed a protocol for use of CBT with forensic patients and systems of staff supervision. Associated research has been undertaken evaluating elements of the CBT programme. This includes group programmes targeting low self-esteem for individuals with psychosis, psycho-education initiatives, and consideration of sense of self, adaptation and recovery in this client group. Though this work is not yet published, it has been aired at a recently convened conference on psychosis in a forensic setting staged at the University of Central Lancashire (Allan and Cawthorne, 2006; Benn and Laithwaite, 2006; Laithwaite, 2006; Walker and Connaughton, 2006).

This conference also saw contributions from researchers at the University of Manchester studying CBT for psychosis and anger in a forensic population (Haddock, 2006), and a call for a new approach to studying the relationship between violence and psychosis (Taylor, 2006). Staff from Ashworth presented work on CBT for forensic patients diagnosed with schizophrenia who are violent (Vishnick *et al.*, 2006). At the same conference, staff at Broadmoor Hospital described their efforts to introduce a comprehensive psychological treatment programme for psychosis (Williams *et al.*, 2006). One of the Carstairs projects is also a collaboration with Rampton Hospital (Benn and Laithwaite, 2006).

All of the four UK high-security hospitals and many lesser secure hospitals have latterly introduced psychosocial interventions of some form or other, and commenced research studies of the same (*see* Allan and Cawthorne, 2006; Benn and Laithwaite, 2006; Laithwaite 2006; Vishnick *et al.*, 2006; Walker and Connaughton, 2006; Williams *et al.*, 2006). Similarly, all of these hospitals have been involved in attempts to engage the workforce in relevant training. For example, a substantial accredited PSI staff training programme has been established at Rampton Hospital under the leadership of Gerry Carton.

A number of training projects have been undertaken at Ashworth over the intervening years that have employed models of whole-team training that bear many of the features described here. The first Ashworth programme was commissioned from external sources in 1999, and further waves of training have followed. More recently, Ashworth has begun to seek accreditation for nursing practice development unit status for wards involved with implementing PSI, and a nurse consultant with the specific role of driving forward psychosocial interventions within the hospital has been appointed. These developments go some way to justify our earlier enthusiasm for these ideas and reinforce the belief that the original Ashworth proposals had sufficient merit to be taken up at the time.

Conclusions

With hindsight, in the light of the recent rush to implement psychosocial interventions within secure care services, including the four UK high-security hospitals, it can probably be stated with confidence that the case for PSI in high-security care has been well and truly made. The fact that the idea of adopting psychosocial approaches into these settings would not now brook any argument is, indeed, a great leap forward from the circumstances we found ourselves in. The equally plain fact remains that the explicit reason for denying us the opportunity to do so, on the basis of questionable transferability of an externally derived evidence base, is still available to contemporary doubters – as it always would have been until someone made a start somewhere.

However, it seems that our position that innovation could run in parallel with research evaluation is now the accepted orthodoxy. Hence, disappointingly, it really would have been a good idea to make a start in Ashworth in 1995. Nobody can predict what might have resulted, but I am left with the disappointing feeling that just possibly, for once, Ashworth could have been in the vanguard of something creative and innovative, with all the potential benefits for patient outcomes, staff morale, and, dare I say it, better public relations.

Those practitioners who have been involved in earlier initiatives might recognise some of what has been described here, and those who are working to implement these ideas and practices currently probably still face some challenges, and deserve full support and goodwill. They are likely to continue to wrestle with issues involved in transforming the context of practice into one primarily defined in terms of care and treatment as opposed to a singular focus on containment. It is to be hoped that the inclusion of the high-security hospitals more closely within the wider NHS structures of management will assist with this, but other trends in the political management of the NHS may equally result in detriment. The practicalities of thoroughly implementing psychosocial approaches raise some difficult-to-resolve questions. For example, what are the implications for user involvement and therapeutic alliances, and what does this really mean in a high-security setting?

Despite the various challenges, psychosocial approaches offer a meaningful way of addressing the criticism that a care and treatment vacuum exists at Ashworth. All of the high-security hospitals are now in a position to address some of this type of critique. I sincerely wish success in these endeavours to all those with a stake in bringing this about. There is, however, always room for a note of caution. The experiences described here beg the question of whether organisational forms, such as large high-security hospitals, will inevitably stifle creativity and practice innovation. Reflection upon the notion that these institutions may serve other social functions, beyond the patient career trajectories of individual detainees, or for that matter the staff who work there, may suggest that all activity is subordinate to containment (of one sort or another). In other words, maybe conservative social control will always be privileged over radical habilitation and rehabilitation for those who are doubly deviant and devalued – mentally disordered offenders.

Our experiences with the hospital's news management machine were, admittedly, a minor irritation, which we shrugged off relatively easily but they possibly speak of a more enduring malaise in the system. The abiding impression was one of an institution with an incredibly low default setting for critical voices, and little sense that out of critique, progress might follow: a peculiar organisational psychopathology of Ashworth.

The 'no news is good news' philosophy might in some way offer insight into the difficulties we had in attempting to enact large-scale practice change, and could continue to pose questions for the complete success of current attempts to implement PSI. With hindsight, could the institution cope with transformative changes? Might that change lead to a discomforting discourse across and beyond the wall, which in some way could threaten its symbolic containment role? If the 'special' hospitals begin to look a lot like any other hospital, do they lose some of their power and mystique in the symbolic order of things? Or put it another way, the institutional isolation previously remarked upon for its stifling and oppressive malignancy, is most purposively undermined by inclusion strategies and service innovation. But, it is this very segregation that feeds and underlines the public and political need for absolute containment of abject criminality (McKeown and Stowell-Smith, 2006).

This might especially be the case if the dominance of psychiatry as a disciplinary power also had its symbolic foundations undermined by extensions of multidisciplinary patterns of working, exposure of some of the inadequacies of the prevailing biomedical model and demonstration of the value of psychosocial care and treatment. One way to resolve such tensions would be to offer the appearance of implementing new practice ideas but to not exactly succeed in completely doing so. A variant of this adaptation to the secure environment is to adulterate the novelty of any approach, to the point that any really transformational change is diluted to oblivion. Either approach would reinvent the status quo. Practitioners concerned with innovation need to be critically aware of these possibilities for resistance to new ideas.

My reflections here may seem like flights of fancy. But it is perhaps a consequence of having personally been involved in struggles and defeats within a total institution that I have developed a heightened sense of fatalism and scepticism regarding possibilities for radical change. When writing this chapter I had cause to approach staff in Ashworth for information that would have allowed me to include more detail regarding recent and contemporary developments. After all, it is now over 10 years since I stopped working there.

I was saddened to find that it was still very difficult to get even the most basic information from staff currently in positions of responsibility for psychosocial approaches in the hospital. Numerous emails and phone calls failed to resolve this. I was not even able to acquire a simple list of initiatives and the dates they were implemented, let alone any more substantial information regarding aims or outcomes. Requests for sight of any unpublished reports or 'grey' material that I could make explicit reference to were pleasantly, but similarly, stonewalled. It seems to me that the tendency towards suspicion and isolation is alive and well.

I want to be proved wrong about Ashworth, as I am generally optimistic about the future of mental health services. Yet if a persuasive case can be made for the large-scale retraction of high-security care (Thomson 2000), then it is likely that psychosocial approaches would be more successful in smaller units. The words of an Ashworth patient regarding the notion of rehabilitation in such settings bear reflecting on in this regard:

> It remains to be seen whether what replaces it is . . . a modern, progressive and successfully rehabilitative regime or whether diminution and closure are in fact the road ahead for the Special Hospitals. My own involvement continues with my detention. I live in hope, but reside in limbo.
>
> (George, 1998, p.106)

One might say that places like Ashworth deserve to be analysed through a cynical or satirical lens, often having all the appearance of a Swiftean dystopia.

One month or so before both Ged and I left the employment of this institution we had a meeting with the director of rehabilitation to discuss the failure of the hospital to implement our project. This senior manager later would occupy a unique position in the history of the NHS. He was to be one of four people simultaneously on the payroll at chief executive salary, though three of them were accommodated thus in states of suspension or 'gardening leave' at the taxpayers' expense.

We faced this manager with our exasperation that the hospital had invested heavily in our education and personal development, but had ultimately baulked at assisting us in putting some of this learning into practice. He, almost comically, but in complete seriousness, stated that, 'if either of you think that you could get a better job elsewhere then why don't you?'. Within the minimum notice period we had both secured offers of alternative employment. I went to work as a lecturer-practitioner between the University of Liverpool and a local mental health trust and Ged left to take up a post as a commissioner of forensic mental health services in Yorkshire. I will leave it to others to decide if these were indeed 'better' jobs.

Even though I have come across some odd experiences in my working life since, I have yet to trump the time I spent at Ashworth. Though my time there was in many ways difficult, and at times quite soul destroying, I also had some good times and was incredibly lucky to have experienced a number of excellent and rewarding professional relationships with patients and colleagues alike. Most obvious amongst these was the opportunity to collaborate with Ged McCann who above all did not deserve to suffer the wrecking of this project.

Jonathan Swift's epigrammatic comment on genius could have been written for Ged, his vision of a psychosocial project within the walls of a high-security hospital and its ultimate fate at the hands of resistive professionals. Paraphrasing Swift (1704) from his *Thoughts on Various Subjects, Moral and Diverting*:

> When a really good idea appears in the world, you may know it by this sign that the dunces are all in a confederacy against it.

The experience of developing ideas and practice regarding psychosocial approaches in a high-security hospital, putting these proposals together, arguing for their implementation, and, ultimately, failing to succeed, was in itself both disappointing and enlightening. At the very least it has informed my subsequent thinking and strategy for similar projects elsewhere. It is also possible that our publications and conference presentations that have covered this territory have in some way assisted others to tread similar ground – hopefully with more success. In the final analysis I am left with mixed feelings about the whole affair.

References

Allan K and Cawthorne C (2006) *Cognitive Behavioural Therapy for Psychosis (adapted for Forensic Settings): a pilot study*. Paper presented at Psychosis in a Forensic Setting Conference, 2 August 2006, University of Central Lancashire, Preston.

Benn A and Laithwaite H (2006) *A Group Programme Targeting Self-esteem in Individuals with Psychosis.* Paper presented at Psychosis in a Forensic Setting Conference, 2 August 2006, University of Central Lancashire, Preston.

Bentall R and Haddock G (2000) Cognitive-behaviour therapy for auditory hallucinations. In: Mercer D, Mason T, McKeown M and McCann G (eds) *Forensic Mental Health Care: a case study approach.* Edinburgh: Churchill Livingstone, pp. 67–75.

Blom-Cooper L, Brown M, Dolan R and Murphy E (1992) *Report of the Committee of Inquiry into Complaints about Ashworth Hospital.* Cm 2028. London: HMSO.

Bustillo J, Laurellio J, Horan W and Keith S (2001) The psychosocial treatment of schizophrenia: an update. *American Journal of Psychiatry* **158**: 163–75.

Chapman P and McKeown M (1994) Taking mental health power for ourselves. *UNISON Health* **May**: 8.

Cooperrider DL and Srivastva S (1987) Appreciative inquiry in organizational life. In: Woodman R and Pasmore W (eds) *Research in Organizational Change and Development* Greenwich, CT: JAI Press, pp. 129–69.

Corrigan P and McCracken S (1995) Psychiatric rehabilitation and staff development: educational and organisational models. *Clinical Psychology Review* **15**: 699–719.

Corrigan P, McCracken S, Edwards M, Kommana S and Simpatico T (1997) Staff training to improve implementation and impact of behavioural rehabilitation programs. *Psychiatric Services* **48**: 1336–8.

Evans N (2000) Working with families of forensic patients. *Nursing Times* **96**: 38.

Ewers P, Bradshaw T, McGovern J and Ewers B (2002) Does training in psychosocial interventions reduce burnout rates in forensic nurses? *Journal of Advanced Nursing* **37**: 470–6.

Ewers P, Leadley K and Kinderman P (2000) Cognitive-behaviour therapy for delusions. In: Mercer D, Mason T, McKeown M and McCann G (eds) *Forensic Mental Health Care: a case study approach.* Edinburgh: Churchill Livingstone, pp. 77–89.

Fadden G (1997) Implementation of family interventions in routine clinical practice following staff training: A major cause for concern. *Journal of Mental Health* **6**: 599–612.

Fallon P, Bluglass R, Edwards B and Daniels G (1999) *Report of the Committee of Inquiry into the Personality Disorder Unit, Ashworth Special Hospital.* Cm 4194. London: Stationery Office.

Finnema E, Louwerens J, Sloof C and van den Bosch R (1996) Expressed emotion on long stay wards. *Journal of Advanced Nursing* **24**: 473–8.

Forster J, Finlayson S, Bentall R *et al.* (2003) The perceived expressed emotion in staff scale. *Journal of Psychiatric and Mental Health Nursing* **10**: 109–17.

Geelan S and Nickford C (1999) A survey of the use of family therapy in medium secure units in England and Wales. *Journal of Forensic Psychiatry* **10**: 317–24.

George S (1998) More than a pound of flesh. In: Mason T and Mercer D (eds) *Critical Perspectives in Forensic Care: inside out.* London: Macmillan, pp. 102–7.

Gournay K and Sandford T (1998) Training for the workforce. In: Brooker C and Repper J (eds) *Serious Mental Health Problems in the Community: policy, practice and research.* London: Baillière Tindall, pp. 291–310.

Haddock G (2006) *Cognitive Behavioural Therapy for Psychosis and Anger in a Forensic Population.* Paper presented at Psychosis in a Forensic Setting Conference, 2 August 2006, University of Central Lancashire, Preston.

Huxley N, Rendall M and Sederer L (2000) Psychosocial treatments in schizophrenia: a review of the past 20 years. *Journal of Nervous and Mental Disease* **188**: 187–201.

Isherwood T, Burns M and Rigby G (2006) A qualitative analysis of the 'management of schizophrenia' within a medium secure service for men with learning disabilities. *Journal of Psychiatric and Mental Health Nursing* **13**: 148–56.

Jubb M and Shanley E (2002) Family involvement: the key to opening locked wards and closed minds. *International Journal of Mental Health Nursing* **11**: 47–53.

Kuipers E (1996) The management of difficult to treat patients with schizophrenia using non-drug therapies. *British Journal of Psychiatry* **169**: 41–51.

Laithwaite H (2006) *Sense of Self, Adaptation and Recovery in Patients with Psychosis in Forensic Settings.* Paper presented at Psychosis in a Forensic Setting Conference, 2 August 2006, University of Central Lancashire, Preston.

Leff J (2000) Commentary. *Advances in Psychiatric Treatment* **6**: 250–1.

Link B and Steuve A (1994) Psychotic symptoms and the violent/illegal behaviour of mental patients compared to community controls. In: Monahan J and Steadman H (eds) *Violence and Mental Disorder: developments in risk assessment.* Chicago: University of Chicago Press, pp 137–59.

Link B and Steuve A (1998) New evidence on the violence risk posed by people with mental illness: on the importance of specifying the timing and the targets of violence. *Archives of General Psychiatry* **55**: 403–4.

MacInnes D (2000) Relatives and informal care givers. In: Chaloner C and Coffey M (eds) *Forensic Mental Health Nursing: current approaches.* Oxford: Blackwell Science, pp. 208–31.

McCann E (2001) Recent developments in psychosocial interventions for people with psychosis. *Issues in Mental Health Nursing* **22**: 99–107.

McCann G and McKeown M (1995) Applying psychosocial interventions within a forensic environment. *Psychiatric Care* **2**: 133–6.

McGuire J (ed.) (1995) *What works: reducing re-offending – guidelines from research and practice.* Chichester: Wiley.

McKeown M and Liebling H (1995) Staff perceptions of illicit drug use within a special hospital. *Journal of Psychiatric and Mental Health Nursing* **2**: 343–50.

McKeown M, McCann G and Forster J (2002) Psychosocial interventions in institutional settings. In: Harris N, Williams S and Bradshaw S (eds) *Psychosocial Interventions for People with Schizophrenia.* Basingstoke: Palgrave, pp. 211–35.

McKeown M and Stowell-Smith M (2006) The comforts of evil: dangerous personalities in high security hospitals and the horror film. In: Mason T (ed.) *Forensic Psychiatry: influences of evil.* New Jersey: Humana Press, pp. 109–34.

Mental Health Nursing Review Team (1994) Working in Partnership: a collaborative approach to care. Report of the Mental Health Nursing Review Team [Butterworth Report]. London: HMSO.

Moore E, Yates M, Mallindine C *et al.* (2002) Expressed emotion in relationships between staff and patients in forensic services: changes in relationship status at 12 month follow-up. *Legal and Criminological Psychology* **7**: 203–18.

O'Carroll M, Rayner L and Young N (2004) Education and training in psychosocial interventions: a survey of Thorn Initiative course leaders. *Psychiatric and Mental Health Nursing* **11**: 602–7.

Rask M and Levander S (2001) Interventions in the nurse–patient relationship in forensic psychiatric nursing care: a Swedish survey. *Journal of Psychiatric and Mental Health Nursing* **8**: 323–33.

Romme M, Honig A, Noorthoorn E and Escher A (1992) Coping with hearing voices: an emancipatory approach. *British Journal of Psychiatry* **161**: 99–103.

Ross R and Fabiano E (1985) *Time to Think: a cognitive model of delinquency prevention and offender rehabilitation.* Johnson City, Tennessee: Institute of Social Sciences and Arts, Inc.

Ross R and Gendreau P (1980). *Effective Correctional Treatment.* Toronto: Butterworths.

Steadman H, Mulvey E and Monahan J (1998) Violence by people discharged from acute psychiatric inpatient facilities and by others in the same neighborhoods. *Archives of General Psychiatry* **55**: 393–401.

Swanson J, Borum R and Swartz M (1996) Psychotic symptoms and disorders and the risk of violent behaviour in the community. *Criminal Behaviour and Mental Health* **6**: 309–29.

Swift J (1704) Thoughts on various subjects, moral and diverting. In: Davis H (ed) (1939) *The Prose Works of Jonathan Swift.* Volume I. Oxford: Basil Blackwell.

Tarrier N, Yusupoff L, Kinney C *et al.* (1998) Randomised controlled trial of intensive cognitive behaviour therapy for patients with chronic schizophrenia. *British Medical Journal* **317**: 303–7.

Taylor J (2006) *The Relationship between Violence and Psychosis: time for a different approach.* Paper presented at Psychosis in a Forensic Setting Conference, 2 August 2006, University of Central Lancashire, Preston.

Taylor L and Jones S (2006) Clinical governance in practice: closing the loop with integrated audit systems. *Journal of Psychiatric and Mental Health Nursing* **13**: 228–33.

Taylor P, Leese M, Williams D *et al.* (1998) Mental disorder and violence. A special (high security) hospital study. *British Journal of Psychiatry* **172**: 218–26.

Thomson L (2000) Management of scizophrenia in conditions of high security. *Advances in Psychiatric Treatment* **6**: 252–60.

Van Humbeeck G, Van Audenhove Ch, Pieters G *et al.* (2001) Expressed emotion in staff–patient relationships: the professionals' and residents' perspectives. *Social Psychiatry and Psychiatric Epidemiology* **36**: 486–92.

Vishnick C, Manson K, Jackson N and Roper L (2006) *Individual Cognitive Behavioural Therapy for Patients with Schizophrenia who are Violent.* Paper presented at Psychosis in a Forensic Setting Conference, 2 August 2006, University of Central Lancashire, Preston.

Walker H (2004) Using psychosocial interventions within a high security hospital. *Nursing Times* **100**: 31.

Walker H and Connaughton J (2006) *Learning Curves: psychoeducation for psychosis.* Paper presented at Psychosis in a Forensic Setting Conference, 2 August 2006, University of Central Lancashire, Preston.

Wessely S, Buchanan A, Reed A and Cutting J (1993) Acting on delusions: I prevalence. *British Journal of Psychiatry* **163**: 68–76.

Whittaker D and Stickley T (2003) Happy families: expressed emotions and team dynamics. *Mental Health Practice* **6**: 34–7.

Willetts L and Leff J (1997) Expressed emotion and schizophrenia: the efficacy of a staff training programme. *Journal of Advanced Nursing* **26**: 1125–33.

Williams E, Wilson C and Dudley A (2006) *Implementation of a Comprehensive Psychological Treatment Programme for Psychosis in a Forensic Setting.* Paper presented at Psychosis in a Forensic Setting Conference, 2 August 2006, University of Central Lancashire, Preston.

Chapter 5

Listening to patients in 'Ashworth time'

Carey Bamber

A recommendation of Blom-Cooper

I worked as Deputy Manager and Development Worker at the newly established Ashworth Citizens Advice Bureau Patients Advocacy Service (ACPAS) from November 1993 to July 1997. The service, initially funded by the Special Hospital Services Authority (SHSA), was the first formal advocacy service to be established in a high-security setting in the UK. A key recommendation of the Blom-Cooper Inquiry (Blom-Cooper *et al.*, 1992), the service aimed to offer Ashworth patients access to independent advocacy, and support to the newly developed Ashworth Hospital Patients' Council. In this chapter, I offer a narrative of my experience of working at Ashworth after Blom-Cooper but before Fallon (Fallon *et al.*, 1999).

The post Blom-Cooper Inquiry Ashworth Hospital in the autumn of 1993 was a place of ambiguity, confusion and possibility. Smarting from the condemnation of a very public public inquiry, my sense was that the hospital community was riven by a lack of clarity over its future direction. It was into this simmering environment that I arrived in November 1993, tasked along with my colleagues, to develop a robust, independent advocacy service for the patient population. At the time the latter stood at approximately 600 people contained across three separate but physically adjacent sites.

The Blom-Cooper Inquiry (Blom-Cooper *et al.*, 1992) had followed the broadcast on Channel 4 in 1991 of the TV exposé, *A Special Hospital*. The programme alleged that there had been a systematic abuse of patients at Ashworth. The documentary alleged that patients were regularly and routinely abused by staff, and that managers were not in control of a staff culture dominated by the Prison Officers' Association (POA). The inquiry panel consisted of experts and was chaired by Sir Louis Blom-Cooper, a judge well known for his experience and skill in public inquiries. He had served as Chair to the Jasmine Beckford Inquiry, as well as numerous other high-profile cases. The inquiry sat between September 1991 and March 1992, with the final report published as a hefty two-volume text in August 1992, containing 90 recommendations. Following publication, a taskforce was established to develop an action plan around the recommendations, and work rapidly began to address some of the key themes identified in the Blom-Cooper report, including the need to change the culture of the hospital and to develop a therapeutic focus.

Its recommendations included the the immediate establishment of a patients' advocacy service which should be 'adequately resourced, independently constituted and managed, with competently trained personnel' (Blom-Cooper *et al.*, 1992).

Why advocacy?

The 1980s had gradually begun to witness mental health service users, survivors and their allies being engaged in developing advocacy in mental health settings, most notably in Canada, Holland and the UK. The main model was of a service led by volunteers, many of whom had had personal experience of mental and emotional distress and who had experience of contact with psychiatric services. The notion of advocacy included support, information and representation to patients. The support builds on the recognition that many people are disempowered in their contacts with and experiences of psychiatric service interventions. Advocates seek to ensure that patients' views are heard and acknowledged in clinical and other decision-making contexts. This is particularly important as most countries employ legislation (such as the Mental Health Act 1983) which allows for the detention of people considered to represent a danger to themselves and/or others, by virtue of their mental disorder. This legislation allows for people to be forcibly treated with medications that may have significant and disabling effects on the person, and also control other aspects of a person's life. In a hospital where patients' daily lives were so hidden from public view, the inquiry recommendation for the establishment of a patient's advocacy service was particularly pertinent and was long overdue.

Initial interest in delivering the one-year contract for the Patients Advocacy Service at Ashworth Hospital was received from MIND (the National Association for Mental Health), The Mental Aftercare Association – MACA (now known as Together), and Knowsley and District Citizens' Advice Bureau. However, at this early stage the hospital management's attempts to impose a 'gagging clause' on the service provider ultimately led to the withdrawal of MIND from the bidding. The contract was won by Citizens' Advice Bureaux (CABx), with the management overseen by an advisory committee that reported to Knowsley and District Citizens' Advice Bureau (CAB).

Whilst CABx had extensive experience of delivering advice services, the foray into formal mental health advocacy, let alone within a secure setting, was new. That said, the national network of CABx had plenty of practical experience of developing advice services in health settings, and within the north had a number of mental health located advice services such as Middlewood in Sheffield, and the mental health services of Salford. In addition, a small, part-time advice service, was already in operation in another high-security hospital, Broadmoor, (as an outreach service of Bracknell CAB), and effectively all of these services were offering a mix of advice and advocacy to patients and, to some degree, staff.

An academic review of advocacy in Ashworth made the point that:

> In negotiating the contract, the most difficult element to resolve was that of confidentiality. The CAB operates within very strict principles and confidentiality policies which do not allow information about a service user,

or information disclosed by a service user to an advocate/advisor, to be shared with a third party except in the most extreme circumstances. Even then, it is only with the permission of senior members of the National Association of Citizens' Advice Bureaux (NACAB). This was unacceptable to the hospital. Therefore, a compromise had to be found to enable the NACAB policy to be maintained as far as possible within the special circumstances which apply in a high security hospital. The NACAB officer involved at that time remembers the hospital trying to be very prescriptive in its demands, and their inability to accept the independent nature of the new service. The review found that echoes of this issue remain today.

(Barnes, 1999, p.46)

The Patients' Advocacy Service contract document drawn up by the SHSA stated that the purpose of the service was:

- to provide a free, impartial, confidential reactive advisory service to individual patients
- to assist those patients in expressing their views, needs and concerns
- to assist patients by representation where appropriate
- to assist the co-ordination and facilitation of the Ashworth Hospital Patients' Council (quoted in Barnes, 1999).

And so, with effect from January 1994, we set out with an initial one-year contract to develop and deliver advocacy in a high-security setting, and began with the recruitment of the core staff team. In advocacy project terms in 1994, the Ashworth CAB Patients' Advocacy Service was probably the best-funded advocacy service in the UK, with a service manager, deputy, three full-time advocates, two part-time administrators and an office suite resplendent with designer fittings and a set-up budget that was the envy of the voluntary sector.

By January 1994, most of the staff team was in place, the office was open, and the Ashworth Hospital Citizens' Advice Bureau Patients Advocacy Service was formally launched – to a cautious reception from staff, but an encouraging wave of interest from the patient community intrigued by the new arrivals. Recruitment of advocates had drawn together an interesting group of people – an experienced psychiatric nurse, a qualified occupational therapist, and a former CAB advisor. Other applicants came from a wide variety of backgrounds, including the clergy, community work, psychology students and a number of existing Ashworth staff. Prior to coming to Ashworth, I too had been working for the CAB, supporting a local mental health sector planning group in Cheshire, as well as running a resettlement project for street homeless people in city centre Manchester. As individuals we were excited by our new roles, and were going to need all our cumulative skill and experience for the task that faced us.

Advocacy in a secure environment

Perhaps the first challenge for the hospital and its new service was clarity over the status of the project staff – employed externally, but needing ready and immediate unescorted access, it was crucial that we were 'key cleared' and trained. This meant all project staff with patient contact undergoing security training, control and restraint training, and signing up to the hospital security procedures which were contained within a hefty set of manuals. In the four years I worked at Ashworth, the service was never furnished with copies of the manuals, despite having committed to maintaining the procedures. Our early security induction included an initiation into the Ashworth Chamber of Horrors – we attended a security talk in a room with a curtained-off wall, which was later theatrically drawn to reveal home-made tools and weapons fashioned from day-to-day items, and discovered in routine security searches or during incidents with patients. Toothbrushes embedded with razor blades, makeshift nooses and garrotes, concealed snooker balls, sharpened polycarbonate knives . . . and all this followed by time in the gym learning how to repel an attack.

For the first time I began to realise that part of the Ashworth culture and mystique was built on preserving, promoting and publicising the dangerousness of the patients – and cultivating a fear of the patient population. While doubtless of concern, this was in stark contrast to my experiences in acute psychiatric services, where people are generally of unknown propensity in terms of dangerousness, and yet are cared for in infinitely less-secure conditions, with far fewer and less-skilled staff. Another victim of this cultural naivety was the newly appointed communications manager. She courted controversy with a comment to the local media in which she described herself as feeling perfectly safe within the provisions of security of the North site, only to be proverbially attacked by a backlash from the staff side which made the front page of the local paper. In those early months we were treated cordially by most staff, although a number of us received warnings from some hospital staff – 'check your car tyres and brakes regularly before leaving the site', 'be careful who you talk to'. We also heard the stories of bullying and victimisation of staff who were seen to side with patients. During the Blom-Cooper Inquiry, we were told that members of staff who were seen to break ranks would be treated with disdain. They had been subjected to intimidation, with windows being smashed, car tyres slashed and excrement posted through letterboxes.

The patient population

In 1993 Ashworth Hospital contained over 600 patients (with a male to female ratio in the region of 6:1). It employed in the region of 1300 staff. Perhaps 90% of the patient population at any one time had arrived at Ashworth through the criminal justice system, having been remanded to conditions of high security or directed to a secure hospital following trial and conviction. The Ashworth catchment of the early 1990s covered the north of England, south to Birmingham, the West Country, North London and Wales, and many patients found themselves a long way from home. Other patients had been transferred as convicted prisoners from prison at the direction of the Home Secretary, or were subject to detention under other lesser used legislation like the Criminal Procedures and Insanity Act which allowed for the detention of those considered unfit to plead or be tried for an offence.

Patients' histories were invariably complex, with all having been judged as presenting a clear and immediate danger to themselves and the public. The notoriety of a small number of patients ensured that the media was always in close proximity, and in the last 20 years the hospital has struggled to stem the flow of confidential papers and information about individual patients that has regularly been leaked and sold by unnamed staff, visitors and others.

While the majority of patients had arrived following contact with the criminal justice system, a small but significant number had not entered Ashworth as a result of contact with the criminal justice system. They had been referred from local services because they were considered too dangerous or difficult to manage, or they needed some form of specialist input. However, there were others whose journeys were even more surprising – and I was shocked to find patients in their early 30s, who had arrived at Moss Side hospital (the original South site) as children and had grown up in conditions of security. At the other end of the age spectrum were a number of extremely frail and aged patients (mainly men). One had spent over 54 years of his adult life in Rampton, Broadmoor and Ashworth following a serious conviction in his late teens.

In terms of diversity, as with most secure mental health settings, Ashworth housed a significant number of patients from black and minority ethnic communities. Much has been written in recent years regarding the over-representation of people from black and minority ethnic communities in psychiatric inpatient settings, and secure services in particular. In the early 1990s only basic attempts had been made by the hospital to address the cultural and spiritual needs of patients from black and minority ethnic groups, although local communities had offered much assistance through the friends and family groups. A local Imam had been appointed who attended for Friday prayers; limited translation and interpreting services were available. During the mid-1990s, as the hospital catering system changed, halal and other culturally appropriate meals became available. The patients' shop began to stock hair and skin products at the request of patients and the Cultural Awareness Group (CAG). The CAG was a patient group facilitated by staff, which met on the North site of the hospital, offering discussion and support and activity, which at one point developed its own band, and organised cultural awareness events across the hospital.

The average length of stay for a high-security patient in the mid-1990s was said to be between 8 and 12 years for patients – although some would come and go very quickly, for example those on remand who may only pass through while being assessed pre- or post-trial. Others would spend the majority of their lives in secure inpatient settings. For those who did move on, outright discharge to the community was almost unheard of. Most patients were required to transfer to conditions of lesser security. A significant percentage of the concerns that were shared with advocates over this period related to delayed discharges, and on some occasions patients would wait years for a bed to become available in a regional secure unit near their home areas, only to find themselves being pipped at the post for the bed as a more acutely ill patient was prioritised over the more stable long-term patient.

For other patients, the transfer dream was quickly shattered, as patients whose mental health had stabilised sufficiently for transfer, and who had enjoyed a degree of freedom within the Ashworth secure perimeter – ground parole and a personal lighter for cigarettes for example – struggled to adapt to the more rigid regime of regional secure services. In such settings, patients found themselves having their shoe laces removed, their accommodation provided in cramped and less private dormitory provision, and with little external access. Some quickly returned distressed and dispirited, and depressed in the knowledge that a second go may be some time off. For others, the opportunity to move on was even more elusive.

As an individual moves up through the inpatient secure system, they gather a reputation of needing more specialised input, and local services can feel unable to manage perceived needs. Furthermore, where those patients are women, the bed spaces become less available as bed numbers reduce. Where patients have specific needs or additional disabilities, the problem gets more difficult. However, since the 1990s, the commissioning arrangements for secure services have shifted to localities, and one of the underlying issues that fundamentally affected transfers has been exposed and unpicked. Patients in high-security services cost their home localities nothing – but once they came back to the locality they were high cost – thus creating a perverse incentive for local services to denounce local connections and attempt to limit their liability for the transfer of patients' continuing care.

The hospital environment

Patient accommodation at Ashworth Hospital in the early 1990s was arranged over 250 acres – established on three main sites, with supplementary staff accommodation and administration and support services located around the campus. The original Moss Side Hospital site was still in use, under the title of 'Ashworth South' when I began my work.

Split from the North and East sites by a public road, the South site existed in some isolation, both culturally and to the hub of the Ashworth North site.

The South site housed a series of wards for women patients, a small unit for men with challenging behaviour and learning disabilities, and, surprisingly to me, a mixed-sex pre-discharge ward. Set behind a once-grand administration block, the South site wards were the poor relation of the North site in terms of patient accommodation – unfit for purpose, unsafe and generally unwelcoming. Patients were housed in single room accommodation, but there was no en suite provision, which in a hospital that still locked people in their rooms from 9 pm at night only meant one thing – slopping out. This was in stark contrast to the more modern North site, where the male patients' accommodation included basic en suite toilet provision and was built in single elevation in a campus-style arrangement, to which patients with 'parole' privileges had extensive access.

On my first visit behind the North site wall (Ashworth North is surrounded by a high wall with a marked overhang) prior to my interview, I vividly recall thinking that if you were going to be committed somewhere, the Ashworth environment, with its campus-like façade, well-maintained and attractive grounds, and extensive facilities, was as good a place as any. This contrasted with the environmental conditions on the South side. Their ground leave extended only to the airing courts at the front of the wards, which were surrounded by secure netted fencing and prison-style gating.

Patients living on the East site fared little better than their counterparts on the South site. Internally described as a medium-security site, the East site in 1993 housed a small number of clinical areas. These were single-storey, barrack-like, square-shaped wards, each with an internal courtyard or airing court. Adjacent to farm land and opening out beyond a 'ha-ha' wall towards the M58, the site was underdeveloped in the early 1990s and operated as a satellite of the South site, from where it was necessary to collect the secure keys required for access. A small patient activity area and some administrative services were also co-located on the site. Gradually between 1994 and 1996, patients from the South site were moved to the East site (eradicating the dreadful practice of slopping out), and two new ward areas and a new hostel-type suite were built on the East.

For the patients living on the South and East sites of the hospital campus, visits to the GP, dental services, patients' library, patients' activity suite, patients' shop and other community facilities generally involved a bus journey from one site to the other, as an agreement with the local parish council precluded Ashworth patients from setting foot on the highways and byways of the nearby town of Maghull. Patient transport, and the state of the hospital bus fleet, came to figure as a significant issue in the business of the Ashworth Hospital Patients' Council, to which I will return shortly.

The patients' day

For some, the patients' day would begin with unlock around 7 am, slopping out (for those patients located on the South site), and after breakfast patients would be transported (by bus or by a secure 'walking bus' arrangement on the North site, known locally as the 'movement') to their planned activity or therapy area. For the men of the North site, there was more ready access to education, sports or workshop activities in the rehab building located on the North site, where many patients had been granted a ground parole status, which allowed them some free movement within the secure perimeter at certain times of the day. For the sports orientated, swimming, gym, football, cricket, bowls, tennis, badminton and other activities were on offer on a rolling programme, provided by a dedicated fitness team. A number of patients were able to join football and cricket teams, which played in local leagues, and there were regular patient–staff competitions.

In the education department located above the workshops in the second floor of the rehabilitation building (locally known as the OER), patients were able to undertake a range of education and training courses from basic literacy through to independent study for Open University undergraduate and postgraduate qualifications. While the education facilities of the North site offered much to the patients of that site, one striking feature that we quickly noted was the cultural tendency to describe the women's education service on the South site as the 'school' – which the 'girls' (the women patients) would attend. When challenged on their use of language, most staff would hide behind a term of endearment rather than acknowledging the infantilising nature of the culture and language that was in common currency across the hospital.

In the workshops suite, male patients were able to access a range of training opportunities including upholstery, radio station concreting, TV and radio repairs, art, pottery and ceramics, vehicle maintenance, metalwork and other services, all run by qualified technical instructors and teachers. Patients from the North site were actively encouraged to participate in meaningful day activity in one or more of these areas, and each patient generally had an activity schedule which detailed their daily routines. For patients on the South and East sites, access to any activity on the North site would begin with a slow and tedious bus transfer, unless they were able to attend one of the small-scale home site-based activities that were developed on the East and South sites.

Also contained within the OER were the patients' library, patients' shop and rehabilitative therapy services – where patients might attend group and individual therapy. A weekly rota of access to the patients' library and the patients' shop was in operation, and patients from across the site would have a weekly visit, allowing them a short amount of time to purchase toiletries, cigarettes, stationery, and order from approved catalogues (for example, Littlewoods) or buy snack food and drinks.

Ashworth was a completely cash-free environment, with patients' money centrally managed through a complex system of requisitions. Patients were 'rewarded' for their co-operation with care plans by the provision of a rewards system, which offered tiered payments as an incentive. 'Rewards' as the system was known, were paid in addition to the social security payments already received by many patients – although patients transferred from prison settings were excluded in law from receipt of state benefits. In this cash-free environment, other items ruled as currency, and when a new patient telephony system (another Blom-Cooper Report recommendation) was developed in the mid-1990s, the telephone cards required became the new cash for trade, along with the ever-popular cigarettes. Run as a contracted-out business, with the profit margins of a corner shop monopoly, the patients' shop was the source of significant frustration for many patients and the subject of lengthy and fraught debate in the patients' council throughout its existence.

The Ashworth Patients' Council

During the 1980s, the voice of people using psychiatric services began to be heard through the development of patients' councils. Built on a successful Dutch model, patients' councils brought patients together with hospital managers, planners, policy makers and others to highlight and address concerns. In the UK, patients' councils had been developed in acute psychiatric settings in a number of major cities, and were under development in other areas.

The patients' council at Ashworth was established in the summer of 1993, and had its own office space in the OER building near the patients' shop, where several of the serving officers (chair and secretary) were allowed to work in jobs of trust. The council office in late 1993 had sufficient space for three people, and access to a stand-alone computer. However, it rapidly became clear that more space was needed and so in 1994 the council moved into a new space in the building. This offered additional desk space, and facilitated the re-establishment of the *Patient Days* magazine. With a full-time patient escort (actually an I grade nurse[1]) known as the patients' council co-ordinator, the serving officers spent time between meetings attending to the business of the council, producing papers

1   I grade is a very senior nursing staff grade, now classed as a modern matron. Basic unqualified staff start at grade A, a ward team leader might be E/F.

and minutes of meetings, and acting on behalf of the wider patient group. I spent roughly half my working week with the council, supporting this activity, and the other half managing an advocacy caseload.

Championed by senior members of the hospital management group, the council had been established in conjunction with the inquiry taskforce, and drew elected representation from the majority of the wards across the three sites. By the time I arrived at Ashworth, the council had already developed a constitution and memorandum of agreement, which were formally accepted by the hospital, which in turn had resourced the council and facilitated its development. In a previously unheard of development, the chair of the patients' council had even participated as a panel member in the interviews for the manager and deputy manager of the ACPAS, and patients were appointed as members of the project advisory group and facilitated in their attendance at meetings in the ACPAS office outside the secure perimeter.

Meeting monthly, patients' representatives would attend an all-day formal meeting session, punctuated by regular breaks and a lengthy but sociable lunch. In between meetings, occasional subgroups would be held, focusing on particular issues. Meetings were supported by a patients' council support team – staff from across a variety of services in the hospital who had been agreed by patients effectively as allies to the process. Topics considered by the council topics were broad and varied. They covered the day-to-day lives and experiences of patients – including the patients' shop, transport, catering, leave from the hospital, delayed discharges, patients' clothing, stores, searches, care and treatment, parole and other privileges, access to psychological therapies, family and other visits, and patients' complaints. Speakers between 1993 and 1997 included the Ashworth chief executives, senior management team members, Dr Richard Williams from the Health Advisory Service, the Right Honourable Paul Boateng, MP (Home Office Minister at the time of the visit), members of the Mental Health Act Commission, Charles Kaye from the SHSA, civil servants from the Department of Health and Home Office, and a range of other visiting dignitaries.

Ashworth was not alone in developing the Patients' Council and Advocacy Services – within months of the establishment of the Ashworth Patients' Council, Broadmoor followed suit, with Rampton shortly afterwards. The development of advocacy took longer, as the hospitals had to tender the projects out. In order to develop communication between the respective councils, I visited both Broadmoor and Rampton councils on a number of occasions, and with the support of the Home Office and the SHSA, we managed to arrange joint visits between members of all the high-security hospital councils. Hosted at Rampton Hospital, patients from Ashworth and Broadmoor Councils were transported across the country to share concerns and common interests in the first meeting of its kind. On another occasion, I joined the chair of the Ashworth Patients' Council on a trip to Broadmoor to view the newly refurbished patients' shop facilities that were provided by Booker Cash and Carry. This was a service where patients were able to pick up a basket and select their items for purchase; a far cry from the cramped, counter-only shop on the Ashworth site.

The patients' shop was a rich vein of complaint from patients, whose access to the external world for basic toiletries, cigarettes, sweets, drinks and other sundry items was non-existent. Run by a private contractor, the shop function was tendered out by the hospital as a going concern, and doubtless was an excellent small business. For the majority of patients who were physically active, the NHS hospital meal provision, which was designed around bed-ridden, short-stay patients, left people still hungry – and the shop was the only other source of relatively accessible food. Patients on their weekly shop would purchase crisps, fizzy drinks, noodles and other snacks to effectively (albeit poorly) supplement their diets. For others, one of the main sources of occupation within the hospital (as with many psychiatric units) was smoking – an expensive habit in a corner shop world – and most patients ended up smoking roll-ups made with cheap pipe tobacco.

Complaints and concern about patients' food, smoking and the shop were regular topics of discussion at the patients' council meetings – with the state of patient transport the runner-up issue. The well-rehearsed food complaints were a major issue, not least because the catering services were built on a per capita allowance designed, as already mentioned, for a short-stay, bed-ridden patient population. Additionally, one of the impacts of neuroleptic medication for some was an increase in appetite – which for this patient group could only be met by whatever snack food they could purchase from the shop or whatever snack provisions wards purchased over and above their allowance.

Another hotly contended issue around food was the lack of culturally appropriate provision for patients – halal meals, for example. The patients' council campaigned hard to secure halal meals – although some patients withdrew their support on discovering that the cost of halal meal provision was higher than the general provision and would be met from the overall budget. For a time the halal meal provision was a more popular option amongst the wider patient community, who considered its quality to be higher, with reputably better meat content. The catering department soon intervened, and only patients attending Friday service were considered eligible for halal meals.

Another bone of contention for patients was hospital transport. As mentioned, patients were moved between sites by bus – and the hospital owned and operated a small fleet of vehicles, including high-security court transfer vehicles, people carriers used to move individual patients on home, hospital or other visits, and a single-decker bus used to move patients between sites for education, therapy, shopping and recreation. Despite the geographic proximity between sites, patients could never be moved intersite, on foot. For those travelling from the South or East sites to the GP surgery on the North, for example, the journey could take upwards of an hour as the bus edged between wards, with radio staff counting patients onto the bus, moving to the next ward and waiting for the next patients to embark. In winter, patients complained of sitting on the freezing smoky bus, as it inched its way around the South and East sites and into the North site vehicle lock, where it would be delayed for security clearance. In the event of an incident on a ward, the movement would be suspended and all transport stopped. This was a frequent occurrence.

The *Patient Days* magazine was another opportunity to promote patients' views and voices. When we arrived at Ashworth, the *Patient Days* magazine had ceased production, and I was asked to try and encourage the former editor to pick up his pen once more and publish. After some negotiation we were able to secure some joint patients' council/*Patient Days* office space, and production of the magazine started up once more. Catering for a wide and diverse audience, the magazine offered interviews with staff and others, poetry and prose submitted by patients, and topical discussion. The magazine won a Koestler award[2] in its first year and produced high-quality copy. Using some of my contacts from my previous work with street homeless people, we managed to build a connection with the *Big Issue* in the North, and received support from the editor and an opportunity to promote positive stories about mental health in a magazine with a far wider circulation.

Providing advocacy

During the first year of operation, the patients' advocacy service was active on every ward in the hospital, and the service very quickly had to establish a way of managing the referrals that came through. Contact with patients was established in a variety of ways – through referral from staff, families and other patients, or directly from patients' approaches to members of ACPAS staff. As keyholders, ACPAS staff had direct and ready access to all wards and hospital areas – and so they were able to access patients quickly. Patients, in turn, were allowed to contact advocates by internal telephone, and were also able to take advantage of a confidential and privileged mail arrangement. This was an extension of the legal privilege reserved for mail to legal advisors and Members of Parliament.

Advocates would have a regular presence on wards, attending ward community meetings, for example, and were proactive visitors to wards where patients were less likely to self-refer for advocacy support and involvement. For many patients, the support required was someone to voice their concerns – and these tended to focus on issues of care and treatment and the future. The focal point for the clinical team tended to be the weekly ward-based (or fortnightly) patient care team meeting, where all the professionals involved in the care of patients would meet together to review patients' progress and plan for the future. Most patients' experience of this weekly meeting was the inconvenience of having one of the communal ward areas taken over by staff for a morning or afternoon – and patient involvement was generally limited to being occasionally summonsed in to hear the considered team view, or frustrated by the failure to get a chance to talk to the clinicians in charge.

Our relationships with patients tended to be long term and ongoing. As we got to know people better, we became more involved in their lives, supporting them through the mental health review tribunal process and in periods of crisis. On occasions patients would request advocacy when they were in seclusion, or when they had been involved in an incident on the ward. On other occasions patients asked for advocates to be present as incidents were unfolding. I recall being called in one Saturday morning when a patient had climbed up onto the roof of a ward, and had refused to come down until he had an advocate present. On such occasions, our role was probably to bear witness, offer reassurance and to support patients, who may have feared a backlash from staff or other patients. With much of my one-to-one advocacy caseload located on the personality disorder unit

2   The Koestler Annual Awards encourage and reward a variety of creative endeavours from men and women held in UK prisons and young offender institutions, and from patients in high-security psychiatric hospitals, young people in secure units and those referred by the probation service (*see* koestlertrust.org.uk).

(PDU), I supported patients through a number of such scenarios. This was especially the case in the period leading up to the absconding of the patient who went on to make allegations of paedophile activity in the unit, and staff complicity in the trade in illicit drugs and alcohol. This complaint triggered the Fallon Inquiry (Fallon *et al.*, 1999).

In the summer of 1995 chasms began to emerge in the veneer of calm across the PDU. The PDU sited on Ashworth North had opened in early 1994, following a recommendation of the Blom-Cooper Inquiry that clinical units should be developed to provide more focused care for patients. The unit brought together patients with a primary diagnosis of personality disorder (categorised under the Mental Health Act 1983 as 'psychopathic disorder'). The development of clinical units heralded the reorganisation of the patient community, with the emergence of a mental illness unit, personality disorder unit and specialist services unit (covering women's services, and the 'challenging behaviour' services).

In practical terms, the PDU clustered together in a series of adjacent wards patients labelled as having a personality disorder, and aimed to work to a therapeutic community model[3]. Led by a consultant psychiatrist who served as the clinical director for the unit, the PDU quickly established a reputation as a difficult and challenging place to work. From what patients told me, the PDU was for many a difficult and threatening place to live. As an advocate working on the PDU, much of my time was spent dealing with patients' complaints – from domestic issues about ward regimes, to the perceived lack of active treatment that many of the patients complained of. The complexity of whether or not personality disorders are treatable was acted out on a daily basis within the unit, where medication was not necessarily effective and talking therapies were in short supply. A number of the patients I worked with were subject to extensive waiting periods (2 years and more) for group therapies recommended by mental health review tribunals, and conditional discharge to conditions of lesser security remained a pipe dream for many caught in what I always thought of as 'Ashworth time' (*see* Chapter 8 by Mark Chandley).

'Ashworth time' represented the suspension of time for patients, and the lack of urgency in delivering effective and dynamic treatment to patients in secure settings. It appeared to me (and others) that there was an unwritten tariff in the psychiatric disposals of many patients. The unwritten tariff was that an implicit minimum sentence was being applied to each patient according to the index offence being judged by staff. This tariff operated alongside the not-uncommon habit (especially within the PDU) of 'ghosting' convicted prisoners nearing the end of their sentences into secure hospital settings; many patients were left watching their lives passing by with no hope of discharge and real rehabilitation.

Incidents began to occur across the unit, although their focus seemed to be Owen ward. There were allegations of bullying and intimidation, thefts, a fire and drunken binges. Tension was high, and in June 1995 a major security incident occurred following a series of detailed searches taking place on Owen. One morning we arrived at work to find the North site effectively shut down, and

---

3 Therapeutic community principles are based upon a collaborative, democratic and deinstitutionalised approach to staff–patient interaction. Highlighting this approach, patients are generally referred to as residents or members of the community. Traditional staff/staff and staff/member hierarchies are replaced by a more liberal, humane and participative culture (taken from www.therapeuticcommunities.org).

Owen ward patients locked in their rooms. We were escorted to the ward, where I and the project manager spent some time trying to calm the patients through the windows of their rooms.

A number of patients had smashed their windows, and others had been forcibly removed from the ward following an incident that had started the previous evening, when a group of patients had refused to return to their rooms. As the day wore on, the search teams began to unearth secreted weapons, security keys, alcohol and a large number of catalogue items and other goods. More patients were dispersed to other wards, and by the end of the day the patients were allowed out of their rooms and into the communal ward areas, which had been made secure. The tension was palpable in the air, and over the next few days things barely improved.

In the days that followed the shut down, one of the most serious incidents in Ashworth's history occurred, when a patient took a psychologist and another patient hostage with a kitchen knife in the library on Owen ward. Distressed and angry at having his visit cancelled, the patient kicked open the kitchen door, secured a knife and ran through the ward to the communal room where he found his hostages. This marked a serious incident response, and the police were brought in to try and talk the patient down, while the remaining staff and patients were removed from the area. As the patient's advocate I was escorted into the secure perimeter and spent an anxious afternoon in the adjoining ward with the displaced patients. The incident was ended without serious physical injury, although for the patient and member of staff taken hostage it must have been the most shocking of experiences.

The resultant internal investigation was never made public, and the findings suppressed within the hospital. Having attended almost all of the confidential post-incident investigation meetings with patients on the ward, what I heard shocked and scared me. Allegations about the complicity of a small number of staff, plus the life-threatening actions of some patients made me feel that no one was safe in the dysfunctional environment. Yet our team was powerless to do anything other than work within the structure, having been forbidden to speak outside the hospital. The horror of Owen only scraped the surface of what was later to be discovered by the Fallon Inquiry across the entire PDU. But despite what had already occurred, the unit was allowed to limp along, albeit under new management.

By the spring of 1997 Ashworth was once more in the grip of a major public inquiry. Shocking allegations about unlawful activity in Ashworth surfaced in a dossier written by a patient from Lawrence ward (described locally as the pre-discharge ward for the PDU). He had absconded while on a shopping trip to Liverpool. The patient had meticulously planned his escape, and managed to get to Holland where he remained for 3 weeks, keeping in contact with the hospital all the while. During this time he maintained that his absconscion was simply a protest to make public his allegations about the hospital. He returned to the hospital after giving himself up, and following a debriefing at which I was present, was transferred to another hospital. He managed to get the dossier to Alice Mahon MP, who immediately raised Parliamentary questions, which eventually led to the announcement of a further public inquiry into Ashworth Hospital. Fallon ensued.

Very quickly all patients were stripped of many of the flexibilities and privileges gained in the previous years – and home computing systems, video recorders and other personal items were removed from patients' rooms and sent to stores. Visiting regulations were tightened, and the opportunity age of Blom-Cooper was well and truly over. After the Owen incidents in the summer of 1995, my own mental health had begun to deteriorate – I was experiencing panic and anxiety symptoms and becoming increasingly depressed. After a lengthy period of sick leave, I came to the conclusion that for my own health I would have to leave. Ashworth had burnt me out. Finally, in the spring of 1997, I began to apply for other jobs and was relieved to secure a job in a local authority in Greater Manchester where I would develop a user-involvement programme. Leaving was incredibly hard. I felt that I was deserting people who despite whatever they had done deserved something better. I also knew that no other job would be as strangely seductive as this.

The personal price

What makes Ashworth so compulsive a place for us? Whether as observers or as those who have spent time working or living there, it is seductive in a strange and inexplicable sense. The notoriety of some of its inhabitants, and the secrecy maintained by a secure wall – made of both bricks and careers – is a heady mix. When I left Ashworth in 1997, my own (admittedly fragile) mental health had suffered long-term damage. I had experienced four years in the life of a toxic institution – during which time the possibilities of the Blom-Cooper era had dissolved into the sordidness uncovered by Fallon. That slide had not merely developed in the short time between the two, but came from the history of the hospital and the patients who entered it. Men with indeterminate sentences and thus nothing to lose, in an environment that buried its secrets, mixed with a handful of staff that no one held to account led to a system failure that destroyed the lives of patients, staff and others.

   Nine years after leaving, I still think of the place and the people. I wonder where people are now. I meet others who were there, and it takes centre place in our conversations. It is the elephant in the room in discussions about the modernisation of mental health services. Since 1997 much has changed – not least Ashworth's entry into mainstream NHS management as it has become part of Mersey Care NHS Trust. I have too little contact to have an informed view on what life is like there now, or what the future holds – but my personal view is that there is no future for, or humanity in, large-scale institutions. No exceptions.

End note

This chapter was written more or less from memory, and I may well have got some things out of order, out of place or even just plain wrong. I hope that in doing so, I have not misled or misinformed anyone.

References

Barnes DK (1999) *Outside Inside*. Durham: Centre for Applied Social Studies, Durham University.

Blom-Cooper L, Brown M, Dolan R and Murphy E (1992) *Report of the Committee of Inquiry into Complaints about Ashworth Hospital.* Cm 2028. London: HMSO.

Fallon P, Bluglass R, Edwards B and Daniels G (1999) *Report of the Committee of Inquiry into the Personality Disorder Unit, Ashworth Special Hospital.* Cm 4194. London: Stationery Office.

Chapter 6

An account of the psychological team in Ashworth Women's Service

Gill Aitken

There has not been significant progress in developing women-sensitive services over the last decade and some evidence suggests hard-won ground is at
risk of being lost.
(Department of Health/National Institute for Mental Health in England
Expert Briefing, Summer 2003)

Introduction

As the last woman patient left Ashworth Women's Service (AWS) in autumn 2003,
I had mixed feelings. I was among those who had argued that too many women
were inappropriately detained at too high levels of security and that the regimes
and environments did not provide empowering therapeutic models of recovery
and rehabilitation. Indeed, over the years AWS had been criticised for providing
'infantilising, demeaning and anti-therapeutic services' to women (Blom-Cooper
et al., 1992). However, I had joined AWS in 2000, in part, to develop a model of
women-centred and empowering psychological provision, and believed that we
had successfully developed a team and model of working to deliver this. So while
I welcomed the marker of social change, I was concerned that a narrow focus on
the closure as *the* positive outcome would mask important learning opportunities.
What had we learned from trying to develop new ways of working during the life
and closure of services like AWS? What had supported and enabled positive
developments and what had been the barriers to such initiatives?

To start to address these questions, below I reflect on my time at AWS between
2000 and 2004. Clearly, these are my personal perspectives and interpretations,
which may or may not be shared by others working in the organisation at the
time. It feels risky to share a personal perspective and describe some of my experiences: 'putting my head above the parapet'. The flip side of this is if I do not risk,
then how can I or others reflect on and learn from our practical engagement with
experiments in organisational change? In my view, while some of these experiences may be specific to Ashworth, many topics and concerns raised in this and
previous chapters are neither unique to AWS nor can they be simply relegated to
the past. Ultimately, my account may or may not resonate with the reader's own
experiences in the 'here and now'. The reader might also judge whether such

experiences can be drawn on as resources and building blocks to support self and others in developing more timely and appropriate gender-sensitive services to women.

Why work in Ashworth Women's Service?

Previous accounts of living or working in secure women's services indicate that damaging and disempowering effects for both patients and staff are likely (Hemmingway *et al.*, 1996; Leibling, 1998; Women in Secure Hospital (WISH), 1999; Aitken and Nobel, 2001). For some workers, the experienced or anticipated costs of becoming visible, through naming the unnameable ('voicing') or undertaking practical action, including publicly supporting others who do voice, has been experienced as very risky. In this personal context, any of us may decide to 'keep our heads down'. Workers who have taken such risks have reported personal distress or trauma. They have been kept out of 'information loops' or found their careers blocked. Some have even opted to leave a profession or a service. Parallel processes have also been reported for service users. Some try to play the 'good girl' in the system or find ways to cut off symbolically or literally. Some have experienced increased distress or have become stuck for years in (different parts of) the system (Parry-Crooke, 2000).

Why have secure women's services developed a reputation for being such harmful environments? I was familiar with the theoretical or political positions which offered different perspectives on this question. Some emphasised the 'pathology' of service users constructed as 'toxic' to the system. Others focused on the outcome of gendered and other forms of social inequality. The dominance of categorical medical and security-driven models of care and risk assessment within secure mental health settings were also present in the critical discourse I encountered.

I was also aware specifically of the marginalisation of psychology as a profession and that even the most well-intentioned person was at risk of becoming seduced by and inured to the damaging effects of the dominant culture of Ashworth. A risk for some, by repute, was simply of being socialised into dominant models of understanding and practice. For others, conformity to the dominant culture was a survival strategy. Others stayed and conformed to an extent in order not to 'abandon' service users. Maybe consciously or unconsciously, they occupied a 'heroine-rescuer' role. Perhaps, less talked about was the pull (i.e. benefits) of working in a 'special' or high-security setting. These included material benefits of enhanced conditions, facilities, pay and possibilities of accelerated career development relative to other settings, as well as the 'kudos' in working with people identified as the 'most dangerous', 'most complex' and/or 'most damaged' in our society.

While passionate about social justice and women's issues previously, I felt the conditions were not right to build on the work of earlier psychologists and allies over the years. So what changed? By 2000, there had been a number of wider UK government policy and strategic initiatives, which in my view offered important external drivers and resources to develop and support the implementation of service improvements.

Nationally, from 1997, there had been a series of consultation exercises on services to women spanning secure, inpatient and community settings. Although a national strategy for women's mental health was expected in 2000, it was not published until 2002, with implementation guidance the following year (Department of Health, 2002, 2003). Reference to 'women' and 'equality' had also started to appear in wider Department of Health directives.

A number of research and practice initiatives relevant to women had been commissioned by that time. These included: a review of secure services for women (Lart *et al.*, 1998); an analysis of women requiring different levels of secure care in the North West and the factors implicated (Shaw *et al.*, 1999; Dolan, 2001); as well as a Department of Health pilot of a three-day training programme for teams working with women across different secure and related settings (*see* Scott and Williams, 2004).

Personally and professionally in the north west of England, I was working within networks of potential allies. In 1998, I co-founded an independent regional multi-agency and sector forum: Women Working with Women (this met on a monthly basis and held bi-annual conferences until 2006). The regional secure commissioning team had named commissioners with responsibility for women, and set up a steering group (2000–2004) to develop, implement and review standards for secure service provision to women (North West Regional Secure Commissioning Standards, 2001b). I was a member of a women's project development group including representatives from Ashworth and Mental Health Services of Salford with the remit to set out a case for a 'one service model' for women (Jones and Aitken, 2001)

At interview, I was assured that the lead psychologist post would have an explicit remit to take a strategic developmental role working out of two trusts. The aim was to cut across traditional organisational and professional boundaries, and to focus on the development of holistic gender-sensitive and appropriate services for women. This was extended to the development and provision of consultancy, supervision and training where appropriate across professional, agency and organisational boundaries.

In the context of the above developments and commitments, I accepted the post as if it were a project. I anticipated that the service would have approximately 2.5 years' lifespan. Would it be possible to develop and support a reflective and empowering women-centred multi-agency and multidisciplinary psychological team? Could that team contribute meaningfully to service improvements, which met the needs of women service users and yet supported staff in the process? Could such a team model its values and share its resources in its relationships with all stakeholders?

I secured external supervision and used it to focus on organisational dynamics and cross-organisational working. I also set up regular meetings with my line managers and enrolled on a Managing in Health and Social Care course to give me some protected time to understand change management. I did not underestimate the challenge of working at Ashworth. However, I felt that these forms of personal support would help me to contain and manage, and even counter, possible damaging effects.

Proposing and implementing change

Before I joined AWS, I heard through informal networks that my feminist reputation had been discussed by some service members. From personal experience, I knew that a number of negative stereotypes were held about 'feminists'. I needed to clearly share what my values and practice were about: social justice for all, the importance of transparency and accountability to one another and a commitment to share resources. I knew that the existing psychology team had experienced difficulties in recruitment and retention and had been operating with vacancies for a while. The team members I had met reported long hours of working, a sense of being overwhelmed and having to focus on crisis- or reactive-led referrals and challenges. I heard their experience of being devalued and criticised by the wider service for their efforts, in spite of the obvious under-resourcing. Also, I was working across two trusts which both provided medium- and low-security services, which held the potential for 'rivalry' around service development and provision.

For years, the need to enhance patients' access to a range of psychological and therapeutic interventions that took account of the diversity of women had been raised (Parry-Crooke, 2000). In the field of mental health, psychology as a profession has striven to establish itself as occupying an expert position, at least on a par with psychiatry. At the same time psychology like psychiatry has been criticised for 'othering' social groups along dimensions of gender, 'race', sexuality, class, and disability (Bondi and Burman, 2001; Fernando, 1995).

Historically, psychology has claimed 'ownership' over psychological assessments and interventions. In the world of forensic mental health services, clinical psychologists have tended to work in NHS settings and forensic psychologists in prisons, although the numbers of the latter in the NHS have increased over the years. Rivalry and competitiveness has been played out between clinical and forensic psychologists over who should provide what, when and where. In the 1980s, specialist medical psychotherapists were recruited into the NHS and high-security system. More recently other professions (e.g. psychiatry, nursing, social work, creative therapies) have formally expanded their roles and ways of working, with the introduction of nurse consultants and consultant psychiatrists in psychotherapy charged within their own professions to take clinical (therapy) leadership roles within organisations. At AWS, two nurse consultants provided sessions into the women's service for brief periods between 2000 and 2004. Irrespective of which profession, to a large extent 'legitimacy' and 'authority' to deliver psychological interventions has largely remained with professions historically employed in the NHS.

Given the above developments, I arranged to meet key individuals, teams and groups as soon as possible within AWS. I wanted to explore our concerns and hopes and the contributions of different parties. Also I hoped to identify barriers and their character. In particular I needed to identify who might be allies in supporting service improvements and the delivery of my role objectives.

First impressions

As I met with different people, I had sense of a shared vision: to provide services which would better meet the needs of women and to be part of a service valued by all stakeholders. However, the vision in practice varied from person to person. Those who took what I saw as social-psychological user-centred approaches, perceived the power base for decision making to be in the domain of psychiatry alongside influential pairings within nursing. This perception was confirmed as I attended a range of meetings as part of my induction process. Whether or not a meeting took place, start and end times, and final decisions about the types of interventions seemed to pivot on the availability and views of key players and professions. When they were not present, meetings could be cancelled or decision making deferred within the wider team. I witnessed how people who voiced views that challenged the status quo could variously be ignored, talked over, or 'put down'. Diversity in expression of views definitely seemed to be neither encouraged nor welcomed.

This was often my personal experience while in the service. On one occasion at a service management team (SMT) meeting, I experienced being criticised, and no one else intervened or spoke up on my behalf. This was not uncommon. I decided to say to the person criticising me that I felt as if I had been attacked and tentatively raised whether or not they were angry about something that I had said. I explicitly said that I had I risked saying this, because I understood it was our SMT leadership responsibility to role model to the rest of the service the value of diversity of perspectives as well as transparent and open communication. To minimise personalising the exchange, I wondered aloud whether the exchange was because we had not had the opportunity as a team to share with one another our values, roles and approaches to the development of the service. In an attempt to take this forward strategically, I said I personally would find a team away day useful. This was later organised with an external facilitator.

However, I did not always speak out. On occasions I decided the time was not right to engage with the 'battle'. At other times I did not want to risk publicly exposing the service or an individual when individuals external to the service representatives were present. To stay quiet could be difficult, particularly when an 'official view' was portrayed as representative of a consensual service view, when this was not my experience or understanding. In such cases, if I could not open up the dialogue in other ways, I always tried after the meeting to meet with the individual who made such statements.

An example of my silence occurred when I was presenting an activity report to the rest of the SMT. A director external to the service was present. I was repeatedly interrupted and criticised on almost every aspect of its content by a member of the SMT. Other service team members kept quiet, many averting their gaze. I experienced that whatever I said in response to the criticisms was not and would not be listened to, as evidenced by the ongoing interruptions. I felt in the presence of someone external to the team that I could not simply suggest at this point that the meeting be stopped to review what was happening. Before I finished presenting the report, the director announced he had to leave. He informed SMT members that if they had anything they wanted him to know to communicate this via myself as he and I were due to meet later. When we met, his first words were . . . 'Forget what we were going to talk about, I want to talk about what just happened . . . you will not be bullied and harassed like that again'.

Such experiences were not unique to me. Psychological team members reported similar ones at some ward and wider service meetings. As a team, we continued to identify strategies to prepare for and deal with such instances. We tried to focus on the issues raised, rather than engaging with personalised or professional attacks. We tried to have a fall-back position, so that if team members felt unable to counter criticisms there and then, they would indicate that queries would be directed to a more appropriate member of the psychological team. We also tried to anticipate potentially difficult encounters in which it would be useful for me to be present.

My experiences occurred against a background of me being employed as a lead psychologist: highly qualified and with a range of strategies of resistance to change already in mind. Mine was a very different power position to that of a woman patient, assistant psychologist or nursing assistant. At times it was difficult for me to hold onto a sense of respect and trust in my relations with some colleagues. I experienced differences in the values and commitments shared in more closed meetings and discussions and the behaviours experienced and witnessed in more open meetings. This was a topic often explored in my own personal supervision.

First steps in implementing specific changes

With the support of the then service development manager, the SMT initially 'signed off' a proposal to review the resources of, and demands on, psychological assessment and therapy services. This included psychology contributions to multidisciplinary working; existing good practice; and the contribution of other professionals and therapists working therapeutically with women.

The review was informed by discussions and feedback from identified key stakeholders. These included professional leads, ward managers, Women in Secure Hospitals, SMT members, patient forum, therapy practitioners and psychologists, and responsible medical officers. I also attended a range of women's service meetings; we updated the status of referrals to psychology and related therapies; and held a psychological team away day. The final report identified key objectives and recommended the introduction of a centralised system for all (neuro)psychological individual and group assessment and therapy. This was to be from pre-admission through to discharge from the service. The proposed mechanisms for this included the introduction of a new referral system and a proposal to develop an integrated psychological (rather than psychology) assessment and therapy team.

In one sense, such proposals do not look particularly contentious. The recommendations intended to rationalise and make effective use of resources through a single entry point referral system. (Neuro)psychologists, therapists and counsellors could come together as a co-ordinated team to enhance equity of access, range of psychological therapies and quality standards for women patients (*see* also Department of Health, 2004). However, such proposals implicitly called into question pre-existing organisational norms. They implied a shift from a medical to a psychosocial model, which took account of the specific needs and contexts of women's lives. Although the SMT collectively agreed to the review, I soon felt undermined.

I received reports that the 'usefulness of such an exercise when direct client work was what the service needed' had been raised and discussed both within and beyond the service. For me this reflected a crisis-led approach, rather than investment in strategic development to increase and sustain capacity over time. Over my period of employment, (copies of) memoranda and letters were variously received by board members, directors and professional line managers before full discussion of concerns with me. It was at such times that my professional and service line managers' commitment to supporting my role was vital. Importantly, I kept my line managers fully informed, as well as psychological team members who might be at the receiving end of reactions to any proposals or implementations of change.

Recruitment

As the review of psychological service provision was in progress, I also needed to recruit into existing vacancies. Advertisements, job descriptions and person specifications were rewritten to emphasise that patients had a range of experiences and needs, and the importance of team diversity and cross-organisational working. We made it explicit that we aspired to be a reflective and dynamic women-centred psychological team in all aspects of our work and relations, and outlined the support and development structures to embed this. This was to communicate clear expectations of any applicant as well as to open ourselves up to questions about how we practised and supported such an approach.

In the first wave of recruitment, clinical and forensic psychologists were targeted, as I would be the only 'qualified' psychologist working half-time in the service. Once two psychologists had been recruited, I felt that as a team we could deliver specific psychological assessments and interventions. This initial emphasis on qualified psychologists was a strategy to counter possible wider service resistance against the later recruitment of those without a traditional professional or secure environment background. In the second year, we recruited a full-time team member from the voluntary sector. This was followed by a range of formalised secondments and short-term contracts, on a varied sessional basis, of other staff from within the women's service (e.g. nursing), forensic directorate (e.g. rehabilitation services) the wider trust (e.g. eating disorders service) and voluntary sector (e.g. women's centre). We also finalised a service-level agreement to the psychological service for a counsellor from a rape and sexual abuse centre. All applicants were informed that, given the national and regional developments, the future of AWS would be time limited.

Developing a psychological team

In parallel to the above developments, I met with other practitioners (potentially) working therapeutically with women. I wanted to explore whether they were interested in being members of a psychological (rather than psychology) team. People shared their experiences of being marginalised. They were uncertain about change and anxious about loss of professional identity. They feared becoming more visible in the service. They also shared practical challenges, such as the amount of time dedicated to therapeutic work.

This generated three possibilities about these individual allied staff members. First was for them to become core members of the team and commit to attend weekly team meetings. The second option was for these practitioners to be 'link' members and to commit to attend team meetings on a monthly basis. The third option was not to formally ally and to review the position at an agreed future date. Whether or not individuals initially signalled interest or commitment, all received minutes of team meetings and were invited to team development and training days. Within the first three months, five practitioners allied with the team.

Early in 2001 our team comprised four members, in 2003 we had 17 team members from a sessional to a full-time basis. By 2001, we had produced the following mission statement:

Mission statement for the psychological team in the AWS

We aim to further develop and consolidate a collaborative and multidisciplinary/agency WS psychological team to provide a range of gender- and culturally appropriate and timely psychological assessment and therapeutic services for women with complex psychosocial needs.

The WS psychological service acknowledges the diversity and strengths of women users and is committed to working collaboratively and in empowering ways with women. This is achieved by taking an informed gendered and cultural perspective when drawing on user- and peer-evaluated clinical, research, educational and training experiences and literature. This to support and promote the socio-psychological well-being of women who are in (or at risk of) contact with secure psychiatric services/criminal justice system.

We tried to promote an ethos of inclusion but also of accountability to one another, to colleagues and to service users. This was formalised in a variety of ways. I introduced weekly team meetings which I made mandatory for those I line managed. This was to provide a structure to improve communication and co-ordination, and to develop as a team. At meetings, time was allocated to discuss challenges and successes of team working and working into the wider service. As the team grew, managerial and clinical supervision was separated out, ensuring that clinical supervisors met the relevant criteria as specified by therapy and professional bodies.

A centralised system of diary keeping and monthly activity records was set up. This was to improve transparency, communication and awareness of what each of us was doing. Activity included assessment and therapeutic sessions, sickness, holidays, training, supervision given and received, production of reports and attendance at meetings internal and external to the service. Cancellations and non-attendance were also reported on, as was an open section for service issues, which affected activity. No team member (including myself) was exempt, and any team member could have sight of the records. These were summarised to form part of the quarterly activity reports back to the SMT. Finally, I recommended that individual team members kept a personal diary of their experiences to encourage reflective practice. Some did this.

From individual and team feedback, and reflections on my own (power) position as lead psychologist, I became more aware that concerns about my own role and availability could impact on the feelings and work of the team. Some members shared with me that at times they did not want to appear distressed in my presence, as I was their line manager. Talking with the team, as a group and individually, we identified an option for monthly group supervision. Attendance was open to all the team (clinicians, support workers and administrators). We agreed that I would not be present at these meetings, and agreed a system with the supervisor for how matters relating to my role would be fed back to me. We also put in place a review process of the usefulness of the supervision to the team.

At the team's development days, we agreed the outcome of the review of the gender appropriateness of assessment tools, agreed minimum standards for reports, and provided training in administering measures. We also addressed evaluation and training in the gender sensitivity of language, and looked at the contribution our reports could make to patient progress. We agreed that all reports be shared with women before distribution to the wider service, and how differences in views would be incorporated.

Emerging tensions and resistance to change

As changes were proposed and introduced, the resistance from parts of the wider women's service mainly reflected historic splitting between individuals and professions who privileged a medical model and those who favoured a more social-psychological model.

Competencies and confidentiality

Shortly after I joined the service, psychology team members started to report that at care team meetings they were increasingly challenged about their competencies and abilities to carry out aspects of their work. At first, the role of assistant psychologists came under scrutiny, and different responsible medical officers 'demanded' that only 'qualified' psychologists should be employed. As we recruited 'qualified' clinical psychologists, these demands changed to the need for forensic psychologists/consultant psychologists to undertake aspects of the work of clinical psychologists. When the first psychological therapist was employed, her competence was questioned because she was not a 'psychologist'. In the Blom-Cooper Report (Blom-Cooper *et al.*, 1992; *see* Chapter 1), substantial evidence documented the marginalisation of even 'qualified' psychologists and a psychological approach to care within the culture of Ashworth. In the light of this cultural history of disrespect about psychology input to patient care, the above complaints were, to my mind, politically motivated not intellectually cogent.

The suspicion around external workers (to the service or to the organisation) was evidenced through the protracted length of time for service level agreements (SLAs) to be signed off by the management team. This applied to psychology (drafted in 1999, but only signed off in 2002) as well as to the voluntary sector (e.g. the Rape and Sexual Abuse Centre). A similar obstructiveness arose in the signing off of the SLA between the service and WISH. By 2002, I became the only professional lead with a split post across two trusts, and in response to questions stated my intention to stay with that way of working. This position was minuted at a SMT meeting as a 'conflict of [organisational] interests'. I responded by referring to the recommendations of the Fallon Report (Fallon *et al.*, 1999) and good practice guidance. I argued that our wider commitment was to improve services to women that reflected their care pathways and transcended organisational boundaries.

Such challenges around competency and confidentiality, to my mind, reflected a range of underlying concerns from interest groups. This included rivalry over perceived ownership and control of psychological therapies and the direction of travel around patient care and risk. Also, there was no recognition that I had ensured (and openly communicated to the wider service) the team's adherence to professional and therapeutic codes of practice, including boundaries of competency. Similarly I had explicitly communicated via the SMT options about the delivery of a limited service, based on the range of competencies and skills of team members, at different points of the recruitment process.

I appreciated that service members, particularly responsible medical officers, wanted the 'best' for 'their' patients. However, this 'best' was often framed within very traditional and narrow hierarchical frameworks. Vivienne-Byrne (2001) has described this process as probably reflecting a concept of 'safe certainty' in working in secure settings, which is based on what is known or what has been historically used. So for example, medication is identified as the treatment of first choice, and cognitive-behaviour therapy is privileged over exploratory and biographical, or explicitly feminist, approaches to psychological therapy. Clinical psychologists are considered safer than counsellors etc. This conservative stance was evident despite critiques of such systems over the years by user groups and research findings about models of care (Vivienne-Byrne, 2001).

Traditionally, professional training has not attended to the peculiar needs of women. In particular little is included about special aspects of working with women survivors of abuse and violence, or retraumatisation of women and secondary traumatisation of workers in working with survivors (*see* also Department of Health, 2002 and 2003). Yet the value (and competency) of workers whose qualities, commitments and experiences are put forward in good practice guidelines (*see* Department of Health, 2003; North West Regional Secure Commissioning Team, 2001b, were considered legitimate to challenge. The challenges were coming from staff whose own training and experiences provided little legitimacy for their position, but their power to challenge was rooted in their traditional position in the institution.

While psychological team members were being questioned, professionals in training who needed to engage in therapeutic activity and whose lines of reporting and accountability were not to the psychological team were not subject to the same scrutiny by the wider service. In my view this scrutiny probably reflected the traditional unequal power relations within secure systems (dominant medical and subordinated psychosocial models, where the subordinated is always under scrutiny). Also, during any change-management process, innovations are often queried whereas the status quo is not.

The main argument from outwith the psychological team was that non-qualified clinical/forensic practitioners could not work with 'such dangerous women' and did not meet Home Office requirements for offence-related work. Such arguments reflected an assumed dichotomy between offence-related work and therapeutic work. At times, care teams demanded that some psychological team members should avoid talking about index offences with women. This assumed that women's offending could be separated from their lives and from therapeutic consideration. But maybe the main message communicated to the staff member was that their competence to work in Ashworth was in doubt.

This is not to say incidents did not occur from which individuals, team members and the service could learn. For example, early-evening sessions had been introduced in response to some individual women's needs. I received a report that safety had been compromised as a therapist had not turned on a light during the course of a session when daylight had started to go. The escorts outside the therapy room were not able to see into the room clearly. This communication was formalised through a written letter and the future of evening sessions placed under threat.

In another incident, a sentence in a report submitted by the psychological team was ambiguous. One interpretation was that the patient had made allegations of sexual abuse in the past. Due to numerous changes in the timing of the care team meeting, neither the therapist nor her supervisor was available to present the report. The care team decided to immediately follow up the matter with the patient, without attempting to contact the therapist or psychological team members first for clarification. The report was also noted to have not been countersigned by the relevant supervisor. In fact it had on the original but this had been cut off in the printing off by a person – outside of the psychological team – who distributed it to the care team.

For me, the above were examples of very hierarchical, authoritarian and petty reactions. There was little face-to-face communication with the individuals concerned at the time, and letters and memoranda went to different senior personnel outside of the service. I tried to understand this lack of norms about ordinary personal relating in the staff culture. Was there such a lack of confidence in the psychological team? Were certain service members trying to protect themselves or the service from possible criticism in the light of the history of inquiries? Did service members want to demonstrate efficiency and compliance with policy to the wider forensic directorate? Irrespective of the above possibilities, in my mind (and for wider psychological team members) the manner and content of the communications were experienced as further attempts to publicly 'expose' or undermine the psychological team.

'The women's best interests'

As the psychological team developed a presence, patients began to self-refer for contact or therapeutic work. However, this was met with resistance from care team members. 'Objective' and 'rational' decisions were given to restrict women's access to our service. A common claim was that it was 'in the woman's best interests not to engage' or it was out of the care team's hands because of security restrictions. Such claims were powerful forms of resistance and a double bind. For us to 'insist' could be framed as working against the women's best interest or as putting the service or woman at risk.

For example, one woman was due for transfer to a lower level of secure care and she had requested to see her previous therapist. At the care team meeting, the majority decision was that therapy might unsettle her and could result in 'problematic' behaviours or incidents. Such incidents would then jeopardise her placement at a lower level of secure care. A 'rest' from therapy was recommended and communicated to the woman.

On another occasion, I received a request from a woman to see her in general hospital, and took this request to the ward manager and care team. Although she was under escort, two main reasons were given for me not to attend. First, the particular Ashworth Hospital security policy covering women's absence from the service was interpreted as not allowing therapy visits. Second, I was informed that the therapy focus we had before her hospitalisation would, in any case, be detrimental to her well-being. As a way forward I reviewed the particular hospital policy, and recommended its revision as it was not originally developed to take account of general hospital stays. I also reassured the care team that I did not intend to undertake the formalised therapy that we had been engaged with, given the context of her hospitalisation. I speculated that the woman's request reflected the importance of continuity of care and a trusting relationship, which could provide her with an opportunity for her to voice and make sense of what had happened to her. It took almost a month to finally meet with her.

Within the psychological team

Tensions were evident not only between the wider service and the psychological team, but also among team members. We had made commitments as a team to work constructively and openly with tensions and differences. Some of these tensions arose out of the differences we brought to the team. We had varied understandings and ways of working informed by different identities and experiences (rooted in class, race, sexual orientation, disability, and faith).

Other tensions arose from meeting the requirements of the wider professional and therapy organising bodies, which set out criteria for who was able to supervise whom. For example, assistant psychologists would need to receive supervision from clinical psychologists on particular aspects of their work. Some team members reported frustration with their personal and professional development opportunities, and felt the team reproduced a hierarchical system in which psychologists were privileged over counsellors. Over time this reduced, as we identified and supported personal and professional development plans for members to access qualifications and training and to develop their roles, and as we expanded the range of therapeutic backgrounds from which team members were recruited.

As funding of external supervision was limited, tensions also arose in access to supervisors who were available from within the wider institution or as part of wider therapy-training courses. In some instances, team members reported that the supervisor seemed not to be alert to the implications of gender and power dynamics at Ashworth. Also, there was a concern from some that their supervisor adopted an expert (distant) rather than a collaborative position. In reaction, team members reported feeling frustrated, angry, resentful and disempowered. Individually, and as a team, we talked through options and the implications for self- and other learning if members simply disengaged without talking with the relevant supervisors about what was happening. Members subsequently reported attending supervision, after which some communicated to the relevant supervisor that they would end their attendance, while others continued.

Team members also held different views about the value and role of standardised measures in assessment and in evaluating therapy shifts. Some members eschewed the use of standardised tools, particularly in the context of many measures being gender neutral or normed on men. Early on in the life of the team, we systematically reviewed all the psychological measures held within the service for their applicability to women and their experiences. We then researched and identified measures that were more relevant to aspects of women's lives, such as surviving and coping with abuse and trauma. We wanted assessment tools that would inform therapy recommendations rather than be simply tools for diagnosis. We also discussed the potential role of standardised measures to develop an evidence base for supporting the need for a range of therapies and how such tools could be used in positive ways to support a model of hope and recovery. This was then supported by training and review in administration, interpretation and report writing. Tensions were ongoing but we were able to agree a common standard for an assessment package and for report writing and protocols for incorporating women's views and sharing of reports.

Closing the service

In this section, I briefly reflect on aspects of the closure of the women's service.

Placement of women

Ashworth took women from a wide-ranging catchment area beyond the immediate North West region. Discussions started with the relevant high- and medium-security services for each woman's originating authority, alongside the relevant commissioning teams and Home Office representatives. Initially, no woman was identified as requiring high-security care. For women originating from the North West, the regional commissioning team and some local trusts had commissioned needs assessment research. This research was to consider placements, service configuration and bed capacity in different parts of the secure system (Shaw et al., 1999; Dolan, 2001; Pidd, 2001). The secure commissioning team set up and facilitated meetings, inviting representation from across the region, particularly the medium-security services and AWS. Up to this time, AWS (alongside Rampton and Broadmoor) had a history of providing women-only services. At lower levels of NHS secure care, the concept of women-only wards or services was still relatively recent.

As discussions about the clinical needs and risk of women and placement options progressed, some AWS staff argued that the existing medium-security services and associated care models could not safely manage or care for a number of women from Ashworth. Profiles and scenarios of needs and risks were presented, followed by heated debates on the implication of different models of care for recovery and rehabilitation and resource demands on services. Some, including me, argued that women could be supported at lower levels of security. This implied more creative project management and a different model of care, with staff development and support structures rather than creating a new type of service (Aitken and Jellicoe-Jones, 2002; Aitken et al., 2003).

Following from these discussions, the secure commissioning team produced a paper on its commissioning intentions, including a pilot process for an enhanced secure service. This was put out to a bidding process to the three trusts that provided medium-security services (North West Regional Secure Commissioning

Team, 2001a). At the same time nationally, the concept of enhanced secure services was taken up with three pilots. What differentiates the admission criteria and models of care for women across high, enhanced secure and medium secure services is still unclear. Although enhanced-secure services are part of medium security, they could become an additional tier of service sitting between high and medium security (*see* Edge, 2006). It should be noted that such a level of service was not proposed and neither does it exist for men.

Some medium-security services felt that they had neither the resources nor the skills to support and work with women, whose complex needs were similar to those outlined in the case scenarios provided by AWS. This was also at a time when some medium-security services identified themselves primarily as services for people diagnosed with severe mental illness, rather than personality disorder. Women in Ashworth often were diagnosed with both or with more than one personality disorder (Aitken and Logan, 2004). Also, the availability of beds in medium-security units is generally problematic, which compounded the problem of patient transfer (*see* Chapter 1).

The outcome was that from a starting position of no woman at Ashworth being identified as requiring conditions of high security, approximately one-third of these women were actually transferred to other high-security services as an interim measure. At the time of writing, in 2006, a number of women are still in such settings. Failure of access to lower levels of security was also at odds with principles of the National Service Framework for Mental Health (Department of Health, 1999); people should be kept in the least-restrictive environment and as close to their homes and families as possible. In response to a request from patients' solicitors, I wrote a statement supporting their claim that risks did not warrant levels of high security, and that with appropriate support and resourcing, potential placements at lower levels of security could and should be found. This was communicated and shared with other professional leads, as well as line managers, before submission.

The appeal was unsuccessful, and it was fed back that from within the service, the psychology service provided the only supporting statement. I heard that the psychiatric view was that transfer to a high-security setting was the safest option for the women in the circumstances. There was little public discussion of the implications and outcomes for women transferred to high-security settings. I heard from a line manager that my production of a support statement was considered by some as being naïve. I was clear that on clinical and risk grounds, no woman required high-security care. I felt that more could have been done to support alternative placements, and that the wider system needed be explicit about, and accountable for, the reasons for the decision to transfer the women to a level of high security. Rather than being naïve, I was simply being transparent about the system failing the women. I would argue that others were being politically expedient and opaque in their preferred decision-making rationale.

The introduction of the concept of 'enhanced secure services' was articulated as being necessary to ensure that the needs of women would be appropriately met. However, in my view what emerged from this practical application was that patients were portrayed as particularly complex and particularly dangerous and particularly demanding. What also followed was that the women could only be managed in particular specialist services by (nursing) staff with the appropriate level of expertise – i.e. those who had worked in high-security services. Further, as models of care and associated workforce plans were being developed for an enhanced service, what I experienced was a retreating back into 'safe certainty'. This was reflected in high levels of ward-based staff being proposed per patient (up to a 4:1 ratio) for observation and management purposes. In my view, this reinforced the notion of staff as experts and having the responsibility for the care and management of women, rather than of developing the quality of relationships between staff and patients and working in empowering ways.

While I was reassured that the initial numbers of women identified in the North West for an enhanced service fell dramatically to less than half a dozen, I believe the damage had been done. The impact of the case scenarios and ensuing discussions was to highlight and expose the apparent lack of skills and deficits in the rest of the system. Not only did this minimise the good practice that was in existence, but it also missed the opportunity to build on the existing skills and resources in the system in collaborative and partnership ways. Creative solutions could have been found by supporting (in developmental and empowering ways) staff in the wider system and working in closer partnership with voluntary and community organisations. Many of these latter organisations have decades of experience of working and supporting women survivors of abuse and violence.

Following the Fallon and Tilt reports (Fallon *et al.*, 1999; Tilt *et al.*, 2000; *see* Chapter 1), part of the reason for both the accelerated discharge programme and the closure of the women's services at Ashworth and Broadmoor (2007) was that the majority of women in high-security services did not present a high risk to the general public, but rather to themselves (WISH, 1999). In this sense, women became commodities or political pawns, as services played out ownership over the direction and control of care and service provision. One-third of the patients were transferred to other high-security settings until enhanced-security services could be commissioned, built and recruited to or beds made available at medium-security levels.

Transfers and follow-ups

Following the closure announcement in 2002, the SMT developed a project plan to transfer patients and re-deploy staff. While plans directed and provided the framework for the proposed stages of closure, the process spilled out into the current care environment. Psychological team members observed and heard from women patients how the latter tried to reassure or provide emotional care to staff (who were uncertain about their own futures). Women reported that they did not want to worry staff with their problems and concerns. Psychological team members were not immune to such anxieties. As a team we articulated commitments that our own anxieties and concerns would be held and processed within the team and via supervision. The intention was not to let this personal work affect relationships with patients. Team members also articulated a commitment to stay unified and cohesive until the last woman left – which was mainly achieved subject to further funding or the ending of contracts.

Some of the patients had been at Ashworth for over 15 years and had developed a range of relationships with other women and staff. From women's accounts, many had experienced little sense of control over their care pathways, which dated back to childhood. They had had many repeated experiences of relationships with others (staff and other patients) ending abruptly or without warning following transfers to different wards and services, as well as the impact of staff absences.

As part of the women's preparation for transfer, psychological team members worked with other staff to run transition groups. For many women, the fear of 'failing' at lower levels of secure care was uppermost in their minds and heightened because the familiar (i.e. Ashworth) would no longer be an option for them in the future. For others, who were going to high-security services as an 'interim' measure, there was the fear of being 'stuck' in another high-security service. Recipient services were invited to attend the groups to answer the women's questions. Group work was supplemented by support sessions for individual women around specific transfer concerns.

More psychological workers were engaged with a number of women in individual therapy. Precise transfer dates were uncertain (or changed at short notice), and therapists and women agreed from when to prepare for each therapy session as possibly the last. Given the number of women to be transferred to Rampton, a day meeting between the psychological teams at both services was arranged. On the day, strategic and operational matters were discussed to build a consensus between the teams.

Over the course of a year the number of wards reduced, in part reflecting staff moving to other services and organisations and in part because of the non-viability of wards or of safety being compromised. There was a consequent pressure on receiving services to take women earlier rather than later. There were instances, when some women were given extremely short notice of their transfer to another institution. At times, this reflected a window of opportunity (bed availability). At other times, care teams reported this to be in the woman's 'best interest' in order to reduce distress and so maintain safety of the service for staff and remaining patients. To my mind, there was little opportunity for many women to have a sense of control over their pathways or to express a range of feelings associated with loss, leaving the familiar or fears and anxieties about the future.

Despite negotiation with women for follow-ups by their therapists (and originally agreed by care teams and receiving services) a number were subsequently stopped. This was most often for women transferred to high-security services at the direction of the receiving clinical teams. We were informed that follow-ups would unsettle the women, who were thought to need time to adjust to the new environment, or that they no longer wanted the follow-up. As we had no direct contact with the women, the team attempted to either challenge or clarify these accounts. We negotiated with the receiving psychology teams to ensure that when this was a receiving service's clinical team decision, this was clearly communicated to the women concerned. Where follow-ups were definitely not going to happen, team members wrote 'ending letters' to the women. This was to mark the end of the therapeutic relationship. It also signalled again the progress made in the therapy, as well as the coping strategies and options identified with the women in the preparation for transfer and hand over of therapeutic work.

The disbanding of the psychological team

Following the closure announcement, staff futures and re-deployment were key concerns for all professional groups and agencies. Initially, as might be expected, the nursing profession, as the largest staff group, was the focus of the organisation's attention. By early 2003, on behalf of the psychological team I submitted a discussion document to human resources outlining options to maintain a women's service psychological team within the trust. I argued that the development of the team was unique. I believed that we had successfully developed a model and framework which could be described as fulfilling the objectives we set out with. I also believed that we modelled commitments of transparency, integrity and sharing of resources with others. The team was also unique in collectively having extensive experience in working with women with a range of needs and risks across community, prison and all levels of secure care settings.

Initially there was a positive response to the paper, but over time we heard nothing. When I pursued progress, I was told that the document could not be found. Team members tried to remain optimistic, but feelings of frustration and anger were experienced, directed outwards to the wider organisation. We prepared for a range of outcomes, including the disbanding of the team. We identified strategies to support us as a team to learn from and also make sense of our contributions, the closure process, and our future employments.

For example, some team members had written into their personal development plans identified time-bound projects to progress particular pieces of work, which would go beyond the closure (e.g. a gender-specific group therapy programme, which could be piloted for women across settings in working with anger). Team away days were held to reflect on and review how we had made a difference and contributed to improved experiences of women in contact with the system. We secured funding for supervision to continue past the actual closure. Strategies for taking the learning experience and development of good practice and thinking into new settings were also talked through. Team members also generated ideas and proposals for a book; to bring together all psychologists who had worked in the service over the years to 'mark the end of an era'; and a proposal for the team to hold a 'follow-up' retreat weekend the following year.

As contracts ended, team members returned to their permanent posts or were re-deployed (to male services), initiatives like the proposed book and meeting up as a whole group were abandoned. This was because members had difficulty in protecting dedicated time or funding, as new or existing services had other priorities.

Summary

In this chapter I have focused on my experience of staff and organisational relations and systems, rather than women patients. Individuals, teams and professional groups hold much of the institutional power to stimulate, support, suppress or sabotage the change needed for social transformation. Often changes to the status quo provoke anxiety and anticipatory loss. Anxiety and fear can solidify into strategies of resistance and destructive relations with one another. It is not simply how we relate to one another as individuals or members of particular professional or social groups, but also the procedures that we put in place to ensure the appropriateness, safety, quality and effectiveness of service provision. The difficulty is that we can develop systems that become too unwieldy and bureaucratic. These can stifle not only forms of creativity and responsiveness but also the cultivation of leadership qualities including supporting, enabling or driving positive change forward. Anyone working or living in secure settings will be aware that time seems to expand exponentially when planning, implementing and evaluating change and progress.

The high-security hospital system performs particular political and practical functions for wider society. As an institution, Ashworth mediated the interests of politicians and the Home Office through its workforce. Its unionised history of the main body of (nursing) staff was rooted in Prison Officers' Association, with its penal and security-driven focus. While its hospital function emphasised the need for models of care and rehabilitation, my view is that the healthcare system itself is rooted in a categorical and medical model creating particular groups (professionals, managers, security experts) who have vested interests in reinforcing and maintaining particular hierarchical and expert structures.

As Pilgrim and Eisenberg (1985) argued, the development of patient-centred services in the high-security system was doomed to failure from the start. Their pessimism indeed might be amplified given the particular political, economic and social situation of women in secure settings (Department of Health, 2003). On the one hand, attempts to introduce innovation risked exposing the inadequacy of the status quo, implied by the critique of Pilgrim and Eisenberg (1985). On the other hand, the closure of the service does not necessarily challenge the status quo if the same systems of thinking and care are maintained in other high-security hospitals or if medium-security units become 'mini-Ashworths'. The closure may have reflected a pragmatic solution to identified political risks or embarrassments, through re-deployment of individuals and groups and reconfiguration of services. In such ways, all become expelled from wider consciousness, as if they had 'never existed'. In this way, organisational and societal amnesia is generated. Since the closure, and following re-deployment, individual team members have fed back their experience of trying to take the thinking, learning and good practice to other services (for both men and women). However, again it is often within a context of marginalised positions and in the absence of a critical mass of allies. From team members' accounts, the resources that they could offer and share in relation to the development of services often do not seem to be held in a wider organisation's consciousness.

For the specific organisation in which the team worked, I am firmly of the view that there was a missed opportunity to build on the resources of the team to benefit the wider organisation in its development of services to women. As far as I am aware, the development of the multi-agency and multidisciplinary psychological team at that time was unique in secure settings. In part the possibility of its development reflected the benefits of working in high-security services and in part the support of professional line managers. In my view, it also reflected the resilience and commitment of the women and men who joined the team at different time points. However, perhaps in the most part it reflected the decision to close the service, so that over the final 16 months energies of the organisation and professionals began to be redirected to more immediate pragmatic issues. These included the pragmatics of developing bids for parts of the service and workforce to become future providers of enhanced secure services to women, for the service to demonstrate safe, timely and financially prudent closure of the service; as well as the re-deployment of a large body of staff.

This is not to say that scrutiny and questioning of psychological practices abated, but in my experience they decreased in intensity and prevalence over time. As the service formally marked its closure with an event for the staff, for me the marginalisation of the contribution of psychological approaches was evident. In the formal acknowledgement of the contributions of individuals and professions to the service over the years, no reference was made to psychological practitioners or approaches

And what did the service do for the patients? As the team developed, I believe the women had access to a greater range of psychological therapies informed by a women-centred and gender-sensitive approach. This was reflected in authentic, transparent and consistent ways of relating by team members, including sharing of reports and attempting to work with tensions which emerged. If a team member cancelled a session, then systems were put in place to ensure the woman received notification by another member of the team, if not by the relevant person. Some women for the first time were able to access a dedicated therapy space off-ward. As a team, we were not able to significantly influence the direction of the women's transfer pathways. However, consistency, continuity and reliability of what was agreed between women patients and their therapists were upheld – if not directly through face-to-face follow-ups, these were communicated in writing.

As a team, we bore witness to the many experiences of the women in aspects of their care pathways into, within and out of AWS. I hold onto the view that sometimes bearing witness is just as important an act as being able to contribute directly to change.

At the time of writing (July 2006), some women from Ashworth are still resident in high-security services. I have seen no public reports of the progress of women transferred to lower levels of secure care. In the North West, up to six beds are identified for women who require enhanced medium-security care. In London the figure stands at 50. In my view, women are still inappropriately detained at too high a level of security and for too long. In part this reflects the absence of appropriate placements at lower levels of security and in the community. As services debate and argue about which diagnostic categories they should utilise or which threshold criteria for accessing community, forensic and secure services should operate, many women continue to be deprived of their liberty wrongly, or they are inappropriately spiralled into secure care.

Acknowledgements

I would like to acknowledge the resilience, strength and resourcefulness of the women patients, a number of whom I was privileged to meet. I also want to acknowledge the commitment, resilience, creativity and support of psychological team members. Thanks, to my line managers who placed a leap of faith in my appointment and who actively and publicly demonstrated their support of my approach and actions on numerous occasions. Thanks also to my supervisor, who enabled me to keep grounded and shared her insights. Thanks to the work and alliance of Women in Secure Hospital, as well as the range of colleagues I met and worked with in and beyond AWS. Whether working in alliance or challenging me, all these groups and individuals have contributed to my thinking, practice and learning.

References

Aitken G and Jellicoe-Jones L (2002) *Individualised Approaches to Care and Treatment of Women with Severe and Enduring Complex Needs.* Unpublished paper submitted to North West Regional Secure Commissioning Team.

Aitken G and Logan C (2004) Dangerous women? A UK response. Women in prison and secure psychiatric settings. *Feminism and Psychology* **14**: 259–62.

Aitken G and Nobel K (2001). Violence and violation: women and secure environments. *Feminist Review* **68**: 68–88.

Aitken G, Pitman I, Jellicoe-Jones L and Thomas A (2003). *Development of North West Regional Secure Women's Services: women's cognitive needs/impairments.* Unpublished discussion paper submitted to the North West Regional Secure Commissioning Team.

Blom-Cooper L, Brown M, Dolan R and Murphy E (1992) *Report of the Committee of Inquiry into Complaints about Ashworth Hospital.* Cm 2028. London: HMSO.

Bondi L and Burman E (2001) Women and mental health: a feminist review. *Feminist Review* **68**: 6–33.

Department of Health (1999) *The National Service Framework for Mental Health – Modern Standards and Service Models.* London: Department of Health.

Department of Health (2002) *Into the Mainstream: gender and women's mental health strategy.* London: Department of Health.

Department of Health (2003) *Mainstreaming Gender and Women's Mental Health: implementation guidance.* London: Department of Health.

Department of Health (2004) *Organising and Delivering Psychological Therapies.* London: Department of Health.

Department of Health/National Institute for Mental Health in England (2003) Expert Briefing. *Women-only and Women-sensitive Mental Health Services.* London: Department of Health

Dolan R (2001) *Feasibility Study of NW Region Secure Commissioning Teams Strategy and Development Plans (for Greater Manchester and Mersey/Cheshire Zones).* Unpublished report submitted to North West Regional Secure Commissioning Team.

Edge D (2006) *Women's Enhanced Medium Secure Services (WEMSS): a scoping exercise for developing a research and evaluation strategy.* Unpublished report commissioned by and submitted to National Oversight Group (NOG).

Fallon P, Bluglass R, Edwards B and Daniels G (1999) *Report of the Committee of Inquiry into the Personality Disorder Unit, Ashworth Special Hospital.* Cm 4194. London: Stationery Office.

Fernando S (ed.) (1995) *Mental Health in a Multi-Ethnic Society: a multidisciplinary handbook.* London: Routledge.

Hemingway C (ed.) (1996) *Special Women? The experience of women in the special hospital system.* Aldershot: Averbury.

Jones L and Aitken G (2001) *Greater Manchester Women's Services: a 'safe and secure' one service model.* Unpublished report on behalf of MHSS/Ashworth Women's Service Project Group submitted to Mental Health Services of Salford Trust.

Lart R, Payne S, Beaumont B, MacDonald G and Mistry T (1998) *Women and Secure Psychiatric Services: a literature review.* Report no, 5, 1998. University of York: NHS Centre for Review and Dissemination.

Liebling H (1998) *Women Abused at Ashworth Special Hospital.* London: Women and Mental Health Forum.

North West Regional Secure Commissioning Team (2001a) *Initial Schemes for Interim Arrangements. Greater Manchester, Merseyside and Cheshire.* Liverpool: NWRSCT.

North West Regional Secure Commissioning Team (2001b) *Standards for Women in Secure Services.* Liverpool: NWRSCT.

Parry-Crooke G (2000) *Good Girls: surviving the secure system: consultation with women in high and medium secure psychiatric settings.* London: WISH.

Pilgrim D and Eisenberg N (1985) Should special hospitals be phased out? *Bulletin of the British Psychological Society* **38**: 181–4.

Pidd F (2001) *Position Papers for the Development of New Secure Services for Women.* Unpublished report commissioned by and submitted to Mental Health Services of Salford Trust Board, Prestwich, Manchester.

Reed J (1994) *Report of the Working Party on High Security and Related Psychiatric Provision, Vol 6, Race, Gender and Equal Opportunities.* London: Department of Health.

Scott S and Williams J (2004) Closing the gap between evidence and practice: the role of training in transforming women's services. In: Jeffcote N and Watson T (eds) *Working Therapeutically with Women in Secure Settings.* London: Jessica Kingsley, pp. 167–79.

Shaw J, Davies J and Morey H (1999) *Secure Needs Assessment in the North West – Summary Findings.* Unpublished report submitted to NHS Executive, NW Regional Office, University of Liverpool.

Tilt R, Perry B, Martin C *et al.* (2000) *Report of the Review of Security at the High Security Hospitals.* London: Department of Health.

Vivienne-Byrne S (2001) What am I doing here? Safety, certainty and expertise in a secure unit. *Family Therapy* **23**: 102–16.

Women in Secure Hospitals (WISH) (1999) *Defining Gender issues – Redefining Women's Services.* Report from Women in Secure Hospitals. London: WISH.

Chapter 7

Working in Ashworth Women's Service

Lorna Jellicoe-Jones

Thinking about entering the system

Ashworth was my first job after my training as a clinical psychologist. 'Are you mad?' This was a fairly common response from psychologists who had worked there, and colleagues and supervisors from within my training course. The anxious doubters were particularly worried about the absurd ambition of trying to build effective therapeutic relationships with clients and staff in such an environment. One colleague suggested that if this was indeed my ambition then I needed to seriously consider help. People also warned that this could be the 'death knell' for my career.

The women's service was seen as particularly fraught and problematic. It was seen as a 'war zone'. Nihilism was offered – it was a service where there was no scope or hope for psychological models or provision. Some suggested it was stepping into an ethically dubious setting (in the light of the public inquiries).

In defence of my sanity, and my subsequent decision to work at Ashworth, it had not been a considered career plan. However, I did have the desire to work with people with severe and enduring mental health problems or in some form of rehabilitation services. To me Ashworth's service remit covered this type of work. This desire followed earlier experience working as an assistant within high-dependency services and, prior to this, with clients with long-term needs within the voluntary sector.

My earlier experiences of community development work (in local communities and with communities within institutions) had shaped an approach that was less individualistic and more social, systemic and political then many orthodox approaches to clinical work. I felt that Ashworth was an opportunity to apply this approach in addition to providing me with the opportunity to contribute to the social responsibility, which I believe we all hold, for offences, and the offenders and victims our society contains.

The anxiety and doubt I experienced about Ashworth, based on colleagues' feedback, proved valuable in clarifying my motivation and expectations of secure service working; expectations which were to be more than fully met. I found anxiety, doubt and mistrust permeated Ashworth at all levels of its functioning, including in the pathways into, and out of, its walls. This emotional and emotive climate seemed to be true for both clients and staff. A number of key processes were salient to me during my recruitment.

First there was the extensive degree of *demonising or labelling of the service* and/or its clients. While this is hardly surprising from a lay perspective, it was just as evident from professionals. The latter, I expected to have a more sophisticated knowledge and understanding of human behaviour and more reflectiveness about their own prejudices, For example, the doubting colleagues I mentioned earlier had few insights about their negativity (especially when they had not worked at Ashworth). This point about blind prejudice appeared to be particularly the case with the women's service, where either the women, the service itself or, most likely, both, were presented as inherently the problem. My experience was of a number of the professionals I spoke to simplisticly 'writing off' Ashworth in the same way in which society 'writes off' its patient population as hopeless and demonic. This process of demonisation seemed to be applied to female even more than male patients.

Secondly, Ashworth was seen as a *dysfunctional historical product with limited scope for change*. Past inquiries and individual stories of negative experiences from the past dominated the discourse. Again this discourse seemed more salient on the female side of the hospital (Blom-Cooper *et al.*, 1992; Potier, 1993).

The above appeared to have led to *nihilism in some and optimism in (a minority of) others*. Was it possible to move on in positive ways or did Ashworth, its staff and its clientele, as society frequently suggests of the latter, 'never really change'? During my recruitment research, I noted that there were psychology colleagues working in Ashworth who did have some more positive views and experiences to share. I wondered how much the damning views of those who had left might reflect other feelings and experiences of anger and powerlessness about Ashworth, and their lack of ability, or opportunity, to address these. I reflected that it was equally possible that those who continued to work there needed to rationalise or delude themselves to justify their position. These split positions of denigration or idealisation of Ashworth ('Ashworth the Centre of Excellence') were evident throughout the hospital and were to emerge as a fundamental challenge for constructive working with both clients and staff.

Taking the leap

I decided to enter the Ashworth system despite (or possibly because of) all the above reflections during my recruitment research. My previous experience with difficult patients had taught me that a discourse about demonised clients frequently indicated genuine difficulties and problems. However, it could also reflect scapegoating, as well as staff defences against feelings of powerlessness, frustration and inadequacy. My experience was also that such 'problems' or demons were *not* always insurmountable. The key issue was often whether investment in such individuals or services should continue, and/or whether this merely served to reinforce or collude with the pathological. In such situations, a less simplistic analysis for me included the possibility of a variety of demons (and angels) and variable service outcomes. There are signs that this more elaborate set of possibilities is now being reflected in government documentation. For example *Into the Mainstream*, the Department of Health's (2002) Strategic Development Guidance for women's mental health care challenges the notions of either women or the staff who care for them as an inherent problem or pathology.

With regard to comments that suggested the stigma and negative status of women's services in Ashworth as qualitatively different from other client groups and services, I did not share this view. My understanding was that while many of the problems or 'demons' referred to may have been more extreme, given the nature of the service and its population, the core underlying psychological processes involved were on a continuum with those represented in other mental health populations, and in the services and agencies that exist to address them, i.e. they may have been quantitatively but not qualitatively different. Having worked effectively with various mental health- and risk-related needs, with various models, and in various institutions and services, I therefore felt I had something to offer.

My experience of recruitment was that it elicited significant anxiety, mistrust and paranoia about both potential clients and colleagues, prior to even entering the service. Based on the experiences and issues highlighted earlier in this section, I felt there would be value, both professionally and personally, in being able to directly question and confront the same through the experience of personally being, and working within, Ashworth. The feedback I had received suggested that this experience would also allow me to address any underlying masochistic work tendencies as underlying my decision making!

Despite having processed these issues over a considerable time period, my final decision to work at Ashworth involved further uncertainty, changing from an initial 'no' to 'yes' over the space of a couple of hours. On reflection, I realised that my initial 'no' response was based on caution and anxiety elicited by the views and feedback from others, and associated concerns about others' judgements of me and my professional career. My subsequent positive response reflected my decision and desire to take risks, based on the points I have outlined here. This was to emerge as a further key theme in working at Ashworth, i.e. decision making and the uncertainty and anxiety it could involve. While my recruitment experience involved flexibility and the opportunity to change one's mind without fear of negative consequences, this was to contrast significantly with experiences in Ashworth; in Ashworth, decision making and its processes and consequences represented a major conflict and tension throughout the system.

Really entering the system

Ashworth had a hospital-wide, week-long induction for all new staff. There were two sessions: one a session co-facilitated by a male patient; the other, the security induction. The former involved a resident discussing various patient forums in the hospital and how patients attempted to have their perspectives and needs heard. I recall the individual being humane, articulate, intelligent and seemingly open to dialogue. The subsequent staff security induction focused on the degree of pathology, dangerousness and untrustworthiness of patients. It culminated in the well-established procedure of displaying the 'wall of weapons' to all staff present. All weapons which had been found in the hospital either acquired or made by (predominantly male) patients were on show, and discussed as evidence of the need for us to 'keep our wits about us' with them (the patients)

While there is an obvious need to ensure staff are aware of actual and risk potential, there appeared to be limited attention to how to integrate this perspective (and the anxieties this display elicited) with the previous perspective provided by one of the said dangerous population. The message conveyed by the 'expert' member of staff appeared to have a much greater impact, judging by colleagues' responses, than that provided by the previous 'dangerous, untrustworthy' incarcerated patient. This split presentation reflected a divided discourse I was to encounter recurrently. Empathy and a credulous therapeutic stance existed alongside distrust and risk minimisation, the latter, in a post-Fallon Inquiry (Fallon *et al.*, 1999) environment, often over-riding the former. Reflections about these tensions could and should have been a key component of induction – but they were absent.

With regard to women's services within the hospital, there was no female patient or staff perspective at the induction. Women's voices and their specific service needs were only discussed in response to my identifying my proposed place of work. This served to elicit the same degree of negativisim and incredulity shown previously by the majority of my colleagues. Women were absent from core hospital business. Alternatively they were deemed to be an inherent problem or pathology for, or when, staff working in women's services highlighted their existence. This, I realised, was also a fairly accurate, if unintentional, representation of the status quo.

My subsequent experience of the women's wards served to both reinforce and challenge the messages I had been given as part of my socialisation into Ashworth. Unlike the training buildings and trust headquarters, for example, the women's service wards suggested a lack of attention and significant neglect. The majority were physically stark, barren, desolate empty shells of buildings. They were old, had limited furniture, and had bare walls, barred doors in many areas, and a goldfish bowl office space. Some of the ward areas had children's stencils of animals on the doorways and walls. The symbolic power of keys was constant. So many doors needed to be constantly locked and unlocked – to go to the kitchen, bathroom, bedrooms, to get things from lockers, to lock/unlock seclusion facilities. In many ways the wards reminded me of pens in cattle markets, where animals wander aimlessly awaiting their fate.

In contrast to this stark and physically secure environment, I came across many members of staff who demonstrated genuine warmth and enthusiasm about their work and the women they cared for. They expressed motivation for psychological input and they discussed the women in the service in a caring, concerned way. Equally, however, they acknowledged conflicting feelings about their work and a range of clinical, service and staff concerns about practice, both past and present. These members of staff were aware of, and subject to, the ongoing negative and dismissive comments about women's services I had experienced. While expressing some anger and injustice about their marginalisation and discrimination, their responses suggested a frequent position of learned helplessness or hopelessness as part of their minority status in Ashworth Women's Services.

I realised that my efforts to resist pre-judgement had failed. I was relieved and maybe shocked at the staff's normal humanity. They were not the monsters they had become in my dreams or as had been represented by many of my colleagues. I considered this to be significant for my future understanding and ability to work with both patients and staff. Both could be represented as monsters of one society or another, with little opportunity for them to have an independent voice or to be heard. Powerlessness and prejudice appeared to have relevance for both staff and patients in the women's service.

The women themselves, while clearly having an identity and status as (demonised) perpetrators, also appeared to have been the victims of monsters. This metaphor came to have considerable validity as I gained further understanding and knowledge of their life experiences before and, for many, within, Ashworth. Many of them were horrendously physically scarred through self-injury. Their bodies were a symbolic representation of the significant psychological scarring or victimisation they had suffered in the past.

One of my most vivid memories is of a young woman I met on my induction to the wards. She was like the walking dead, with her wounds, her emaciated appearance, her pallor and her difficulties approaching the staff office. She died during my time at Ashworth, as her body was no longer able to tolerate the injury inflicted on it. Staff described her as a very bright, capable, articulate and assertive, albeit angry young woman, on entering services. She was subsequently equally described as difficult, dangerous and manipulative with the need for high levels of observation and monitoring. My initial responses to this, no doubt like many before me, focused on the need to try to address 'what went wrong'. This was, however, with awareness of a likely range of 'wrongs', at a range of levels and with the likelihood of any change taking considerable time.

In relation to the above experience, I was also aware that Ashworth was not the only mental health service, or indeed system, to have difficulty engaging with women (or any service users) who might question or challenge it. Such difficulties indeed appear to represent a key theme for women being referred up the system (Stafford, 1999; Parry-Crooke *et al.*, 2000). When patients are challenging to the most coercive part of the system, the consequence can be at their most dramatic, as her death demonstrated.

Few of the women were willing, or had the opportunity, to speak to me directly on my initial visit. However, their bodies served to communicate a great deal. As with the other covert lessons I had learnt as part of my induction, this message reflected an additional accurate reflection of the character of the women's service.

Being in the system

Looking back on Ashworth, the above early impressions remain vivid. So too do the following experiences of subsequently working on the wards as a clinical psychologist.

Group work on the personality disorder ward: the tension of security and therapy

One of the four women's wards was a ward predominantly for women with a primary diagnosis of personality disorder. It had about a dozen women living on it. I saw some of the women for therapy and some staff for individual clinical supervision and I attended some care team meetings. Following one very serious incident, in which a number of staff were injured and a number of women secluded, I suggested a group-based intervention to discuss the issues with the women involved as a community. This was based on evidence of the women's abilities to communicate with each other; the lack of attention to the impact of the event on wider ward dynamics and relationships (on a ward where relational security was a key need), and ongoing conflicting messages about different individuals' roles and responsibilities in the incident. Seclusion, containment and management of the women represented the main intervention in response to this type of incident. However, difficulties increasingly emerged in identifying criteria for reducing such interventions, and there was gradual recognition that their prolonged usage was increasing the distress and anger of patients.

My suggestion was initially rejected as too dangerous. Concerns were expressed that the women would be unable to cope and that the situation would culminate in further incidents. Staff also expressed considerable anxiety about their ability to keep control in such a group setting. There was a view that it was better to continue with graded seclusion and management plans focusing on the use of medication, keeping women on observations and/or separate from other 'trouble makers'. I cannot recall where, or how, this shifted to allow the group intervention to occur. It may have been that the traditional formula proved too demanding of staff time, or that some sense was seen about the need for the women to communicate about an important event. I also recall that staff who had, understandably, been very angry with the women felt that the latter had been punished sufficiently. The ward manager eventually supported group sessions going ahead.

While some of the concerns identified by staff were clearly understandable, given the women's relational and emotional needs, the level of anxiety which existed around the group and its occurrence was overwhelming. The whole ward was shut down and women not involved in the incident were moved out of the main ward area. Extra, predominantly male, staff were brought in and sat observing, just outside the main ward area. All staff on duty sat in on the group and there was attention to checking that all alarms were working and response teams were aware.

The group was not easy to facilitate for all of the above reasons. Also the women had other sources of anxiety. These included fearing the consequences of what they said for their relationships with others, and additional consequences from staff and others, including about their degree of liberty. Staff responses on the ward had clearly also conveyed fears about the possible consequences of this intervention and the women's ability to cope with it.

Despite the above, it was possible to hold four sessions with the women involved and staff, and to explore some of the key factors involved. These included certain dynamics within the women and staff, how the women coped with these, and factors which determined their ways of coping. These discussions centred on trust, peer relationships and feelings of anger towards others and their sources. There were no incidents during the groups and the women were able to question and challenge each other to various degrees. The level of staff input (or observation) at the times of the group sessions gradually reduced and they were generally seen to have been positive. The group work was also linked to individual work with named staff, particularly as group discussions were difficult in this context and for women with such needs and anxieties.

Further to this, I had discussions with ward staff about an ongoing community group. This offered a low-key opportunity to discuss community relationships and events, both positive and difficult. It was proposed as a way of proactively developing and reinforcing the women's coping and problem-solving skills and of reducing the risk of incidents. Despite the previous positive group sessions, there remained a number of obstacles to such work. Staff expressed anxiety and uncertainty about the value of this, with a general view that it would be safer, and therefore better, to 'just do activities with them' or nothing. The women themselves expressed a similar reluctance about the proposed group. They feared that peers or staff might misuse information or 'what would or could happen' (in terms of others' feared negative responses).

Some of this group work did eventually begin as a pilot, with a focus on small-group work and activities, and low-key exploration of trust and communication concerns. It was, however, decided not to continue it, after a number of weeks and following a review, as not all women were engaging. The inconsistency in attendance was contributing to additional ward dynamics and staff were not consistently available to encourage attendance and support the work.

This work did, however, highlight specific concerns from the women about the process and procedures of seclusion and re-integration on the ward. This included discussions of ward dynamics and anxieties about being on and coming off observations. This led to a more focused piece of work with the women, which WISH (Women in Special Hospitals) was also eventually involved in, on seclusion policies and procedures. The women also contributed to the design of new seclusion facilities.

In addition to various clinical and policy matters emerging in the group, it elicited anxieties for staff, some of which might have reflected their feelings about the patients and some their equal fear of potentially losing responsibility and control. Staff anxieties and concerns were presented as clinically appropriate and caring concerns to maintain the safety and well-being of all. However, I thought they clearly reflected and served to reinforce the women's dependency and their internalised views of themselves as incapable agents. This work therefore perhaps best highlighted the previously mentioned security and therapy tensions and the ongoing challenges of integrating the two to achieve clinical and risk progress. The previous inquiry's (Blom-Cooper *et al.*, 1992) comments about Ashworth Women's Service as an infantilising regime were noted. While there may have been number of positive steps forward in women's service practice, the underlying infantilisation seemed endemic and incorrigible.

On a more positive note, I was involved in some requested group work on another ward, where patients and staff were experiencing difficulties with a patient with cognitive problems who was being bullied. The staff requested some opportunity to explore these issues with the women. The victim of the bullying did not attend but was informed that some intervention was being undertaken to prevent further bullying, and she was given additional individual support. This group work was experienced as positive in that a number of women expressed anger and frustration, including regarding their powerlessness in their status on the ward compared to staff.

The group did not, as some staff again feared, result in increased problems or risk incidents with the women. It did, however, highlight that many staff had similar negative feelings regarding the patient which they had not disclosed, but which were covertly serving to reinforce the women's bullying responses. The women appeared to be frequently acting out many of the feelings and fantasies of staff. Attempts were made to address this individually with staff to achieve a wider system response, and to address the narrow pathologising of the women as only and always 'the problem'. Efforts were made in such work to normalise and draw parallels in feelings across staff and patients. However, distrust and anxiety created a recurring institutional dynamic. They formed a significant obstacle to staff emotional expression and personal disclosure, regardless of role and status. Other factors were also relevant to staff disclosure, as will be discussed below.

Ashworth Women's Forum: user involvement or containment?

The Ashworth Women's Forum was a monthly off-ward meeting, open to all patients. Its aim was to enable the women to have more of a voice about service needs and developments; to 'empower' women patients.

The forum developed through some interested staff, including myself, joining up with WISH (an independent voluntary sector project which provides various forms of support and advocacy to women in secure service settings). The intention of the forum was to try to create a space for the women, with these aims of support and advocacy in mind. Women were able to declare what they liked and disliked about the service. We invited external agencies to provide information and feedback on certain issues and we identified pathways and strategies to raise women's needs and concerns across the hospital. We also held some social events, at the women's request, to provide both business and pleasure opportunities for them.

Given the history and concerns about disempowerment of women within Ashworth, a key question would be to identify the criteria for success of the forum. Some women did attend; we had an average attendance of four to five women which represented just under 10% of the population. Other women attended on a more occasional basis. The forum continued for over two years during my time at Ashworth, and I understand that it went from strength to strength after I left. There were no incidents of aggression or self-injury during forum meetings, despite some occasional intense debates and discussions. The women raised various service concerns including: access to sanitary wear in seclusion; seclusion processes; food and diet; negative practices on wards; access to activities and leave within the hospital. These were taken up with various degrees of success. We also held some social events. However, these involved some considerable challenges to address the risk and safety concerns raised by certain staff. For example, they feared the negative effects of different women mixing with people from outside the service or each other. The staff expressed worries about aggression, manipulation and bullying. They also feared that the patients might learn negative behaviours from each other and that they might conspire against staff. There was a notable lack of focus by many staff on the potential positive opportunities of such a forum.

In facilitating the forum, additional obstacles and resistances were encountered which were understood to be a consequence of the anxieties and concerns raised by staff. Women would turn up late or not at all due to the ward not arranging escorts. They would have other activities arranged at the time of the forum. The women's desire to attend the forum was minimised or pathologised ('they only want to go to criticise staff'; 'they've got their own agendas'; 'they're not really interested as they never do anything'). Funding for activities was also last minute with no dedicated budget, and dependent on other parts of the service. Feedback on concerns raised by the women was provided but this frequently involved considerable delays, a need for follow-up, or acknowledgement of the concerns but a lack of motivation to consider change. Staff also expressed concerns that the forum was 'anti-staff' and therefore a problem. (It was decided by the women that the forum would be facilitated by off-ward staff and WISH. The service decided on the need for one clinical staff member in attendance for safety reasons.)

My view, in the context of all of the above, was that the forum was a success but that this was largely despite, rather than because of, the wider service commitment. The various difficulties and obstacles that occurred were, in my experience, no different from those experienced in many mental health services, when any genuine attempt is made about user involvement. The service users' voice and power are experienced as a threat to staff and they generate requests for change. When such change is proposed, in an environment which predominantly focuses on risk, security and patient (and staff) control, staff will be threatened. However, in my view, resistance following the experience of this understandable threat is still not acceptable. As in many mental health services, our failure, in the forum was in our neglecting to address and facilitate the obligation of the staff to support true user involvement.

Normal and pathological emotion

Another significant theme I recall from Ashworth relates specifically to emotional expression. Who and what was expected as 'the norm' about emotions, and whose definitions of emotional normality predominated were often bones of contention. The norms on the personality disorder diagnosis ward, for example, seemed to be determined by the system's fears surrounding emotional expression and the need to avoid the same (by staff or patients). Group work undertaken to address bullying within the service had further highlighted staff's overt dismissal or avoidance of their own emotional responses towards the women. In the women's forum staff had articulated similar concerns about the women expressing their independent feelings and needs, even when these were to be channelled in a safe, controlled (but not medicalised or pathologised) environment.

Anxieties about safe, constructive emotional coping and responses are understandable in the context of a high-security hospital and the population it contains. Many of the individuals placed in high security have obviously adopted ways of coping which have been, in different ways, destructive and damaging to others and themselves. Equally though these ways of behaving or coping have been understood as the only remaining survival strategies for those who experience repeated victimisation in a society or culture that fails to recognise fully the extent and impact of abuse (Edwards, 1986; Showalter, 1987; Blom-Cooper *et al.*, 1992; Potier, 1993). The tendency at Ashworth was to evade reflection on institutional or contextual impacts on behaviour and to focus only on the pathology of the victim. This is despite evidence highlighting the role of the unexamined pathology of the hospital triggering re-enactment of many of the experiences underlying many women's risk and offending behaviour (Jennings, 1994).

Evidence of interventions within Ashworth suggested they were frequently aimed at, or focused on, superficial control and containment of the women, predominantly to meet the emotional needs of the system or staff. Such interventions (enforced medication, seclusion, restraint, observations), as has been highlighted in previous inquiries (and in the recent Department of Health *Into the Mainstream* guidance (2002), have frequently resulted in powerlessness, dismissal, invalidation, silencing or marginalisation of female patients. These negative outcomes repeated the patients' experience of previous abusive victimisation. These outcomes were anti-therapeutic and they maintained an oppressive institutional culture.

In addition to the practices and responses outlined earlier in this section, women who became angry and upset within Ashworth frequently received medication or physical containment as a first response. Their anger, grief or distress about past traumas, or such traumas being re-enacted within the service, continued to be diagnosed or pathologised, and further reinforced by legitimised institutional practices. Women were consequently overtly, and covertly, discouraged from acknowledging or expressing emotions due to the feared, or actual, responses which they learned that such expression would elicit.

I also felt this conclusion could be applied to the staff . One, longstanding, member of staff within the service discussed her unwillingness to acknowledge and explore her feelings about her work. She feared that 'once I've started I might not be able to stop or cope'. In this she referred to a range of feelings about the women, her work with them and the system overall. Other staff discussed a desire to try to 'block it [emotion] all out' as it could be 'too much'. Staff's dismissal of any personal emotional responses to, or problems with, the patient who was bullied further appeared to reflect their views and concerns about being a proper professional. One criterion of the latter was of not being emotionally affected by patients.

A number of my experiences within Ashworth suggested that this avoidance or dismissal of any emotional responses to patients particularly focused on any caring, concerned or empathic response. By contrast, feelings of anger and frustration with patients were acknowledged (although denied to have any impact on intervention). Feelings of care, concern or distress about patient experiences appeared to represent a particular threat or pathology. They were to be avoided at all costs by the staff.

I recall one occasion when I became tearful when reading a very powerful poem written by a patient. This was a very controlled minimal response which was acknowledged and rationalised with the patient as evidence of her powerful ability to communicate her experiences. I was subsequently questioned by the ward manager about my well-being, my emotional involvement and my supervision. This was in the context of a lack of, or limited number of, such questions, to staff who made negative critical comments or responses to the women, for example following incidents, or in response to various staff frustrations.

On a second occasion, when I was leaving the service, I undertook an ending session in a seclusion room observed by three members of staff. The session was emotional for me and the patient. She had been able to express her considerable distress in a safe, constructive way. On leaving the seclusion room, I became aware that two of the three members of staff were also tearful. They were able to discuss their distress at seeing the woman in such pain in such an environment.

However, their main concern was to 'pull themselves together'. They did not want to let anyone know they had reacted in this way, due to concerns about their perceived role and ability.

Finally, after I left Ashworth I was invited back to a women's forum event. I planned to attend this as an appropriate boundaried occasion to see the women. I was subsequently informed, however, that certain staff had concerns about the possibly distressing impact of my visit on some women. My motivation for wanting to attend was also questioned as possibly reflecting some over-involvement, particularly in the context of my having shown distress on leaving the service.

Responses to the expression, or attempted expression, of different emotions within the women's service are not unique to Ashworth. While they may be more overt and extreme, they are seen to be consistent with (and reflective of) wider cultural and gendered expectations and responses regarding emotional expression, and regarding madness and the need for social control (Ussher, 1991). However, the position of women at Ashworth can be seen as damned three times over, given that they are *female* offender patients – they are women, they are offenders and they are mentally disordered. This triple deviance makes it easier to justify a suppressive response in a coercive context of maximum security.

Ussher (1991), for example, outlines gendered models of emotional expression and the unacceptability of women expressing anger or aggression. Feminist writings have focused on how women are socialised to internalise their own feelings and needs, and to have a predominant role and identity in caring for the feelings and needs of others. Chesler (1972) and Mitchell (1974) highlighted the ways in which women are socialised to meet gendered expectations and norms and the role of this in maintaining a patriarchal status quo. Within such models and frameworks, some of the responses and interventions engaged in in Ashworth can be understood as being quantitatively, as opposed to qualitatively, different from those adopted within other institutions or sectors of society.

The above models are also considered to provide an understanding of the system's degree of acceptance, or failure to confront, staff's feelings of anger and frustration with the women. Such feelings, for example, frequently served to elicit and maintain the various socially controlling and dismissive responses towards the women and consequently the power positions and roles of staff engaging in them. In contrast, other emotional responses which suggested some shared staff/patient experience, empathy or support could be a threat. Shared emotional expression and authenticity might threaten boundaries, roles, and power positions. This threat also provokes the dismissal of staff empathy and emotional expression, unless that expression reinforces, rather than destabilises, norms of control (hence the expression of angry criticism is considered acceptable).

Angry patients and empathic or sympathetic staff clearly represented key threats to be monitored, controlled or removed. Perhaps one of the most significant ways in which these were achieved was via the paranoia which was endemic to work within Ashworth.

Endemic paranoia in Ashworth

As outlined above, themes of anxiety and distrust emerged as key prior to my actually having begun work in Ashworth. This is, perhaps, not surprising in an environment inhabited by patients who have significant difficulties in inter-personal relationships, with many of these, from a psychological perspective, proposed to be linked to abusive and disruptive earlier attachments. Psychodynamic perspectives on the clinical needs of such patients, and the impact of caring for them, have, for example, usefully focused on how such inter-personal difficulties or dynamics are re-enacted in systems such as Ashworth (Adshead, 1998; Hinshelwood and Skogstad, 2000)).

It might have been expected, therefore, that issues of anxiety and distrust would have been a consistent reflective focus in all areas of service provision. I have highlighted how, in my experience, this was generally to the contrary. Specific examples have been given of how, and where, this was overcome. But these initiatives (such as the women's forum) and occasional staff emotional dis-cussion or reflection on risk taking were the exception that proved the rule or highlighted the institutional norm. They occurred despite, not because, of over-riding service and system models. They necessarily involved, persistent and consistent questioning and challenging (of oneself and others). They involved having to weather or contain negative feelings from others, especially overt and covert threats in reaction to any move to disrupt the status quo. These negative reactions were paranoid in character – distrustful, critical and hostile to change but, from my experience, driven by intense anxiety.

It is difficult to convey the extent of this anxiety to those unfamiliar with the culture of Ashworth, the distrust it creates and the punishment meted out to those who challenge the status quo. Anxiety within Ashworth was, for me, not associated primarily with patients' behaviour. It was much more about dealing with the anxiety of the institution, which was embodied in the negative reactions of certain colleagues to efforts at therapeutic progress. As outlined above, this could result in the various dismissive or controlling responses the women expe-rienced. These staff responses had equal potential, and actual, power to silence me as well as patients. Attempts to explore and draw parallels between such experiences for staff, including myself, and the women, were very difficult. Such attempts created more of the same dynamic – more distrust and negative responses from certain colleagues. I could find myself in a paranoid spiral.

A confirmatory example of what I experienced as 'endemic paranoia' occurred just after leaving Ashworth. I completed a clinical report and reflected that it had felt significantly easier to write than ones in Ashworth. Further reflection on what had been different identified a primary lack of concern in my new work context about potential negative, persecutory and personalised interpretations of my writing by others. In the new setting I did not fear their reactions. I realised that these anxieties on my part, as much as the clinical content, were key in determining the information I produced for colleagues in Ashworth. While I had developed some awareness of this within Ashworth, it was not until leaving and entering a somewhat healthier system, that I realised the nature and extent to which I had become desensitised to these feelings and internalised them as a cul-tural (and personal) norm.

As with the other points raised in this chapter, I do not consider this point about persecutory institutional systems to be unique to Ashworth. I equally do not consider such processes as self-questioning and challenging, reviews of service and therapeutic goals and expectations, and the containment of negative and high levels of emotion as pathological, or as inappropriate for a clinical psychologist. I have, however, attempted to highlight some of the contextual issues that contributed to these being *particular and extreme* challenges within Ashworth, and their associated particular and extreme impact on staff attempting to work with them.

What did I learn and would I return?

My core beliefs and expectations of my role and opportunities within Ashworth Women's Services did not qualitatively change. I have outlined experiences which confirm my view that Ashworth shares the challenges and problems of other mental health services with female clients. Parallels between the institution and society's responses to women were also reinforced. Parallel processes were evident layer on layer. Ashworth being demonised avoids our scrutiny of wider society. The women's service being demonised avoids our scrutiny of Ashworth. The female patients being demonised avoids our scrutiny of the staff culture in the women's service.

My focus on quantitative as opposed to qualitative differences in Ashworth should not be read as me minimising the problems I encountered about the peculiarities of the women's service and its impact on patients. But a discourse of qualitative difference too readily elides into justifying why things have to be different in Ashworth. In this elision, the place is framed as a 'special' hospital with peculiar residents. In turn this justifies not applying frames of reference from elsewhere. This logic risks closing off Ashworth just as much as other forms of isolation discussed in Chapter 1. Moreover, the quantitative extremes I have discussed do aim to highlight the extreme conditions for female patients in Ashworth, compared to male patients and to women in open mental health services. On a continuum, extremes *ipso facto* have an extreme character.

With regard to my ability to cope with and survive Ashworth, my experiences within the service did involve significant attention to history and the role and status of psychology within women's services. I found this emphasis on context particularly useful in understanding and coping with interprofessional difficulties and dynamics. This contextualising of interprofessional relationships did not aim to dismiss or minimise the difficulties experienced, in the same way that clinical attempts to provide a context or history of the women patients' lives and behaviours does not aim to minimise or dismiss their difficulties. My aim in both was to provide some framework for understanding and intervening as a psychologist, a professional and an individual in an organisation which needed to have a memory.

This did, however, present challenges for my role and identity. Was it possible, in the context of history, to effectively combine being a psychologist and a member of the women's service and to achieve respect and credibility in both arenas? This represented a consistent challenge, particularly in a system where fragmentation and splitting of good and bad identities permeated at all levels. I spent the majority of my working hours within the women's service. With the exception of departmental meetings, the psychological services staff within women's services had limited contact with the majority of psychology colleagues working in the male service.

Wider hospital forums and discussions could involve subjective conflicts regarding my identity and 'family loyalty' to the women's service. Staff from the latter would frequently refer to the service as an intense, dysfunctional family. But there was, as with other more dynamic or systemic analyses, limited opportunity to reflect on, or apply these perspectives consistently at a service level. My recollection is of frequent conflict and fragility regarding my identity as a psychologist or member of women's service staff, with the need to confront and contain the additional source of anxiety this could elicit. However, I saw this predicament as a useful further parallel with the needs of the women, and their attempts to make sense of who, and how, they were expected to be.

Feedback from women's service staff before and on my departure from Ashworth suggested I had had some success in positively integrating my professional and service identities. This felt particularly positive in the context of my having had to raise and struggle with the significant practice and service concerns I have outlined. The fact that this affirmation came from a number of nursing colleagues was particularly gratifying.

When I consider entering and leaving Ashworth and whether I would ever decide to return there, some further key issues come to mind. Prior to entering Ashworth, time and honesty were given to me by my colleagues. Although tainted by the prejudice I noted at the outset, I felt that flexibility and frankness were there for me in the context of decision making. But the women's service I was about to leave felt different. The latter was fraught with key conflicts around power and control and fear of their loss. There was evidence of decision making being frequently avoided through various rearranged meetings or discussions, proposed needs for additional information, and/or absences of key members of staff .

When decisions were made in the daily routines of Ashworth life, they tended to involve a lack of flexibility. Flexibility was seen as weakness and vulnerability and was associated with the core fears of a loss of control. Loss of control was a recurring preoccupation as I have outlined. Fear of its loss meant additional anticipatory anxiety and it prompted tried and tested forms of risk (and thus anxiety) minimisation. In turn, these responses maintained a paranoid stance – threat was all around and hostility to change and suspicion of those desiring it were common. Any actual loss of control warranted blame and criticism (of patients and staff risk takers).

My overall conclusions regarding my time and work at Ashworth were that progress and opportunities to implement alternative ways of working were possible and did achieve some success. This success was built on by those who continued to work in the service after me.

Women's services, however, consistently appeared to be involved in a no-win game regarding their role and status in the hospital. Where there was evidence of success, progress, or increased articulation of the services' needs and rights, the service was criticised and denigrated as being too privileged. When progress was not made, this confirmed traditional nihilism and the demonisation of female patients.

This perhaps reflects the final parallel between Ashworth's Women's Service and the status and position of women outside its walls. As Broverman and his colleagues noted in 1970 and Ussher (1991) reinforces, female patients who conform to societal expectations of dependency, submissiveness and passivity are likely to receive the depressed or anxious diagnoses. Those who do not conform, for example, and who may be promiscuous and assertive or aggressive are vulnerable to becoming 'borderline'. Women, Ussher (1991) argues, are therefore pathologised and cannot win whatever their status. The Department of Health, Women's Strategic Development Guidance (2002) has emphasised the need to consider wider societal gender issues and expectations and how these may be acknowledged and addressed in mental health services and their responses to women. Without this emphasis the anti-therapeutic aspects of the service I experienced at Ashworth will continue to be reproduced at all levels of mental health service provision for women. High-security services will, because of their nature, reflect an exaggeration of this anti-therapeutic trend. However, when those services are scapegoated, we are witness to a defence against our own (society's) fears of change and our (lack of) willingness to confront our prejudices.

References

Adshead G (1998) Psychiatric staff as attachment figures: understanding management problems in psychiatric settings in the light of attachment theory. *British Journal of Psychiatry* **172**: 64–9.

Blom-Cooper L, Brown M, Dolan R and Murphy E (1992) *Report of the Committee of Inquiry into Complaints about Ashworth Hospital.* Cm 2028. London: HMSO.

Broverman I K, Broverman DM, Clarkson FE, Rosenkrantz PS and Vogel SR (1970) Sex-role stereotypes and clinical judgements of mental health. *Journal of Consulting and Clinical Psychology* **34**: 1–7.

Chesler P (1972) *Women and Madness.* New York: Doubleday.

Department of Health (2002) *Women's Mental Health: into the mainstream – strategic development of mental health care for women.* London: Department of Health.

Edwards S (1986) Neither mad nor bad: the female violent offender reassessed. *Women's Studies International Forum* **19**: 79–87.

Fallon P, Bluglass R, Edwards B and Daniels G (1999) *Report of the Committee of Inquiry into the Personality Disorder Unit, Ashworth Special Hospital.* Cm 4194. London: Stationery Office.

Hinshelwood RD and Skogstad W (eds) (2000) *Observing Organizations, Anxiety, Defense and Culture in Health Care.* London: Routledge.

Jennings A (1994) On being invisible in the mental health system. *The Journal of Mental Health Administration* **21**: 374–87.

Mitchell J (1974) *Psychoanalysis and Feminism.* London: Allen Lane.

Parry-Crooke G, Oliver C and Newton J (2000) *Good Girls: surviving the secure system – a consultation with women in high and medium secure psychiatric settings.* London: University of North London.

Potier M (1993) Giving evidence: women's lives in Ashworth Maximum Security Psychiatric Hospital. *Feminism and Psychology* **3**: 335–47.

Showalter E (1987) *The Female Malady: women, madness and English culture 1830–1980.* London: Virago.

Stafford P (1999) *Defining Gender Issues: redefining women's services.* London: WISH.

Ussher J (1991) *Women's Madness: misogyny or mental illness?* London: Harvester Wheatsheaf.

Chapter 8

Ashworth time

Mark Chandley

> This place is strange. It's got its own reality, it's like nothing else. It's sort of just off centre of reality . . . I will tell you, it's difficult reconciling that we are called 'nurses', it certainly is not what I would call a nursing role.
>
> (ward staff member in participant observation)

Introduction

This chapter has been inspired by a PhD I completed recently on the same subject. My own history at and before Ashworth is relevant to understanding how the research was started and the stance I took within it.

I start with this autobiographical acknowledgement before moving on to explaining to those new to the topic 'social conceptions of temporality' (socio-temporality). The chapter is littered with quotes from patients and those nurses who work on the wards. The general theme is to simply ask; how does a person on the wards make sense of time? Particularly when detention is measured in decades and every aspect of one's life has the potential for being interpreted psychiatrically. Then this is overlaid with a need to live with others as a collective whereby a single, dominant timetable applies to everyone. Everyone eats, takes tablets, has workshops and sleeps to the same pattern. All these issues are discussed as some of the temporal issues that impact on the patient are explored. This is followed by recommendations and conclusions relating to this particular view of the world. These recommendations are almost exclusively temporal and represent a beginning to the publication of a new different view of this psychiatrised world.

Autobiographical relevance

The biography, the social situation and temporality will be seen to be connected. One cannot deconstruct the world to separate the phenomena and explore them under strictly controlled laboratory conditions. It follows that social inquiry takes this into account and usually rejects the notion that one can separate the inquirer from the social context. The researcher, the author, the scribe is therefore central to the 'story' and held up for inspection as part of the overall ethnography. Any ethnography recognises this relationship of the researcher to the social data.

Qualitative research does not usually claim 'objectivity' but takes steps to be explicit about the exact relationship of the researcher and then inform the reader – a version of 'reflexivity' (Taylor and White, 2000).

It is critical that the reader be clear that the ethnographic narrative is anchored in a social history and that this departure point is obvious, so that he or she can understand both the social position of the author and his world view and thus contextualise the literature. It is particularly important in this text as the author does not follow popularised explanations. Otherwise the 'story' hangs, mid-air, without any particular context or understanding of its origins. It is as Davies puts it, 'what developed in classic ethnographic texts was the inclusion of some sort of arrival story to give authenticity to the findings' (Davies, 1999, p.11). It is to that end that the author offers himself up for inspection in a kind of brief confessional biography.

I was nurtured in a working class family and lived, for large part, in inner-city Liverpool. My family seemed to resent my chosen path, preferring for me a more unsavoury course, which meant sailing closer to the breaking of the law than studying. For example, learning to access the electric meter was one important 'rite of passage' at 11 years of age. In the longer term, an understanding of the intricacies of sickness and disability benefit were markers of shrewdness and would attract respect. Family 'elders' could be approached on any number of matters surrounding this subject. A cognisance of this craft could not be found in texts but was ground in a common stock of knowledge that was taken for granted and part of everyday life. Simple family rationales explained us as being righteous and upstanding.

One component of the extended family where, even by our norms, petty criminals, involved in an array of minor infractions and crimes though these activities was still understood in positive moral terms, as gaining a living. While law abiding, these infractions were rationalised away as legitimate. Some members of the extended family had various mental illnesses and some had morals that would have my current middle-class cohort labelling them as deviants and 'undesirables'. Many of my former school friends from inner-city Liverpool are 'addicts' or criminals or both. I observe many similarities between clinical notes and my own biography, particularly in terms of the sharing of the same working-class background. It is only the occurrence of semi-informed moral decisions in one's early development that governed whether one made choices to go into crime or reject it. It seems also that nobody is immune from mental disorder, and in some ways it is for the grace of God that you or I have not suffered the same plight as some of the patients I discuss. I do not claim originality here, many of my nurse colleagues and patients share the same working-class origins.

My former family marked me out as deviant. Experience of at least believing one has been different (deviant to others) allows one to be aware that a similar disposal to other deviants was possible, particularly as, as previously stated, my childhood years often do not deviate from common threads in many clinical histories. I worked on many jobs both casual and more formal before starting at Ashworth as a nursing assistant.

Things I have seen do not raise my emotions, only raise an urge to seek explanations. What I don't understand has driven me to study it. I could be described by a simple observer as a middle-aged, middle-class, white male. I work as a charge nurse on the wards at Ashworth Special Hospital. Having worked there for over 20 years I have seen many changes and experienced various accounts of my professional life and of the lives of patients. Some accounts of my world have claimed more authority than others, though few have been written by members of my world. Researchers have spent many hours on wards, but never years and have never 'gone native'. All have influenced to different degrees the daily life on the wards. Additionally, the people on the wards are often 'discounted' in various ways; not least their conceptions of their world have never been voiced.

Ashworth is an unusual setting. It is intimidating to the unfamiliar visitor and an enigma to many who have been there for years. Ward conversation is often laced with coarse and lewd terms. Official language conveys an acquiescence to official policy. Official hospital brochures are glossy and the vocabulary has a caring theme. On my first day at Ashworth, a senior manager proudly claimed that Ashworth was like a 'village'. I fear he had misunderstood a criticism by an outside consultant as a compliment and repeated it, claiming it as a virtue for the rest of his career.

My interest in time goes back to the lyrics of a song by Pink Floyd (1974) entitled 'Time' and its various conceptions of time. However, I could not have begun to study time on the wards without the experience of being employed on them, for a long time. The mere genesis of questioning would not have arisen in the same way if I had taken a traditional route and become a manager. I would have asked different questions from a different view. I also acknowledge that I am still 'native' to the research field and have an allegiance to those on the ward. I have long-held views due, in part, to my cultural position. This study has forced me to examine those propositions, but at the same time my culture has facilitated this study. I have come to reflect quizzically on this notion of culture during my research. While I and others on the wards (including patients) are constantly reminded of our 'culture' by those off the ward, the latter appear to believe that they are culturally abstinent, sterile and beyond the influences of such phenomena.

Long experience has had me question views about 'those on the wards', in how we on the wards are represented through a variety of accounts that are elevated to claim the 'truth'. Those accounts are typically owned by people who do not live or work on the ward, but are often self-proclaimed experts. I want to explore another view of the ward world as accounted for by 'those on the wards'. I also want to focus on time as a means of theorising the situation in a high-security hospital. A focus on temporality or more specifically socio-temporality was borne out of the above history, and a personal observation in which psychiatry has never, not once, been lost for an explanation for any situation. I would argue that psychiatry should have a credible opponent, and that temporal theory is a useful resource in this regard.

The topic of temporality was influenced by participating in a world that, while taken for granted, only required one to step back to see its peculiarities. For example, some patients appeared to retain the fashion of the time their incarceration began. It was as if time had stopped on admission. These people also continued to listen to the music of the same period and most patients reminisced to the period pre-incarceration. Remarkably, most patients would and still do use few daily clock-defined benchmarks. But they would frequently know to the minute, the hour and date that they arrived at Ashworth. I pondered what the differences might be between Terry Waite's (1993) 'without limit of time' detainment, as a hostage, and the same broad situation as a patient in Ashworth. An array of these ponderings, of which the above are merely examples, influenced my choice of study.

A view from the wards

Time is an important commodity in forensic mental health. However, to my knowledge it has never been the subject of any study in a peculiar context, where time is often traded in decades. Brokers of time (clinicians) have not researched the idea of socially experienced time, even though it features so heavily in a secure hospital. I chose also to study facets of 'time' for a first degree thesis and remained intrigued by it. I wanted to study more of the same. I suppose on reflection, I was also frustrated with my own inability to explain, with any legitimacy, the differences between what I observed in my own working experience and how that experience was officially explained on my behalf.

I was working with people who had been incarcerated for decades and who had no definite date for release. The significance of the birthday had been displaced by the importance of the mental health review tribunal (commonly referred to as the 'MHRT') and their only aim being discharge. They seemed to consider discharge to be a rebirth, a type of reincarnation. Neither have patients often wanted my gift of therapy – only to be officially defined as, 'lacking insight and being non-compliant'. Conversely, by their own definition, they were often 'not sick' in the first place. They also explain that handicrafts, cookery and joinery etc (examples of therapies routinely on offer) do not constitute true therapy. The word 'therapy' is ubiquitous and can be applied to any activity. Their experience did not accord with mantras in the official Ashworth newsletters. Men (ward staff and patients) got old and sometimes died. Some patients wanted to stay and often said they 'only wanted to leave in a black bag'. I have seen people grow old and their bodies change shape and their hair become grey. I am not being emotive here, merely reporting.

Additionally, I have persistently witnessed psychiatric interpretation anchoring the world to order inside Ashworth (*see* Chapters 2 and 3 by Mason and Richman). Every legitimate meaning is derived from this departure point. One can of course theorise in other ways, but these theories have no official currency and are therefore irrelevant to official explanations. It is with this departure that I merely want to tell a version of a world that is rarely, if ever, told, at least not by those who 'belong'.

Many of Goffman's (1961) assertions about total institutions are still observable on the wards, though there are many facets that I do not and have never recognised in the field, certainly as he had described them. External stakeholders though have often cited Goffman's text as a mantra, to blindly describe Ashworth wards. Goffman's, *Asylums*, derived from a state institution in the US in the mid-1950s, is assumed, by those ignorant of experience of ward life, to be a literal ethnography of a *present* social situation in Ashworth. However, there are swathes of difference. For example, I have noticed that ward-based staff complain often that, 'we do not count', that 'we are nothing here', that they are 'non-persons' or that they are depicted as 'subhuman' by those off the ward. Staff and patient transcripts are indistinguishable in this regard.

I also notice that when ward-based staff and patients describe the organisation, they frequently agree on many key features. I notice relations between patients and ward-based staff as more gracious and respectful and there is commonly more rapport than has been described by Goffman or beyond. This is the social situation today. In fact, as those called 'patients' and those called 'staff' live together over decades, their view of the world amalgamates into a single culture. The latter has its own stock of shared knowledge, beliefs and norms.

Both patients and ward-based staff complain of being stigmatised and that they are a single lower class of citizen. On the one hand the organisation does not include those on the wards in its own organisational chart (the purpose of an organisational chart is two-fold, firstly to mark out divisions of labour and secondly to map out official relations). Nursing staff and patients symbolically find themselves below the bottom of these charts in that 'subhuman' category that is a collective view on the wards. One nurse stated that while he was waiting for a signature in an office block there were a number of office staff looking out the window at nurses going off duty. To the amusement of office colleagues one said 'there go the arse wipers', reinforcing that lowly social status of the ward nurse.

Furthermore, the Blom-Cooper Inquiry (Blom-Cooper *et al.*, 1992) stained all nurses on the wards of the special hospital and Fallon (Fallon *et al.*, 1999) did the same for the patients. Both ward staff and patients continue with the burden of those two inquiries and of accounts of the ward by those who offer alien accounts (versions of reality that do not coincide with the social experience of those present). While, for example, the local newsletter (*Trust Matters*) reports hand shaking and congratulatory themes, nurses on the wards and patients both report a shared feeling of being an underclass, stigmatised and disregarded. This is the author's world, defined organisationally as an 'arse wiper'.

In temporal terms there is a common sense of 'growing old together', as patients and nursing staff notice body shape changing over the long passage of time. Both patients and nurses on the wards are best explained as one group, 'those belonging to the wards'. This single group considers that they are not related to the organisation. Below the organisational chart and socially isolated, the common explanations of their social situation are akin to Gouldner's (1954) mine.

There were several important features to this study of a gypsum mine in the US. One was that those working above the mine considered themselves more 'cultured' (more refined) than those below and they maintained a social distance. Those down the mine complained vehemently that those above the mine could never understand the dangers underground. The miners would also only work for a good foreman, who had to fulfil particular criteria to attain that status. Those on the wards recognise these phenomena exactly. They use the metaphor of the 'mine' to describe the ward and even go as far as to talk about the effect on the eyesight, most noticeable when one leaves at the end of a shift. Little natural light penetrates parts of the ward, and one is required to squint to see properly when exposed, after many hours, to the sunlight.

Decades of time in isolation on the wards have a single ward culture emerging. This also means that time itself should have special meaning in Ashworth. Time is after all a fundamental category of both understanding and theorising in the world in general.

An overview of socio-temporal theories

It is with this focus in mind that the chapter now concentrates on 'time'. It is notable that the terms 'time' and 'temporality' are used interchangeably in this text. I utilise some key literature to mark out the elemental theory. The aim is to take the reader on a short educational excursion, starting with the forefathers of socio-temporal theory, through to the theories with direct relevance to the social situation in a secure hospital Socio-temporal theory is being used here to offer up a different means of examining the world – as an alternative to the psychiatrised world.

The special significance of temporality

> I am doing time.
> >   (patient in participant observation)

Temporality is an important issue when detained for many years without either any certain future or any estimated date of release (EDR). 'Time' in Ashworth has a special significance. There are several rudimentary reasons that this might be so and these include the following:

- the spans of time involved
- time as a commodity of Ashworth business
- the isolation entailed in detention
- the patient focus on discharge out of 'the system'
- no EDR.

Patients do not generally want to be 'detained', they often do not want the 'care' of 'locks and keys' and nor do they see themselves as patients. According to my research, patients typically value either discharge or to remain in Ashworth until they die. This quote from a patient is not untypical. There is a degree of pre-dictability and a crude career to discharge.

> It's easier in prison. If you can get yourself on the 'block' you don't see anyone. You know what's going to happen and there are no idiots about to fuck you up. It's easy. You have your breakfast banged up, go to the gym, bang up, have your dinner. Gym again, then bang up for tea. The rest of the night is your own. You can lie there and listen to the radio.
> >   (patient)

This sort of message was reiterated by patients frequently. They almost always preferred the predictable cycles, the definite 'sentence', and valued the fixed marker of the EDR. Prison compared favourably, despite the 'perks' of living in a 'hospital'.

In prison, temporal order and length of stay are clear and marked out in rules regarding expected behaviour according to participants. Patients argue that Ashworth is more akin to a prison than a hospital, and from the use of argot on the wards and the collective perception of nurses as 'screws', then this might be a plausible argument. Add in the perimeter and other security, and a visitor could be forgiven for confusing the place completely with a prison. Nevertheless, there are significant symbols of health care – the masses of healthcare professionals, the use of healthcare language and the fact that the hospital is now part of Mersey Care NHS Trust.

Beyond these features one could not talk of time without noticing that many people are detained for decades under the Mental Health Act (1983). These people unusually, have 'time in abundance'. Most of us have a dearth of time and must rush between various commitments, competing timetables and various schedules.

The socio-temporal basis of temporal knowledge

My research took as its departure theories from many academic authors including Sorokin and Merton (1937), Moore (1963), Roth (1963), Gurvitch (1964), Durkheim (1976) and Zerubavel (1979). This academic departure and my passion to tell the story of the little man (hence the importance of the biography) is where the research starts and is maintained. The authors' collective posture of setting society as the focus of speculation is a core concept adopted in this text. These academic forefathers grounded their theories in a fundamental level of knowledge. Key principles underpin essential theoretical speculation and are widely considered as general truths and the basis of theory building. Durkheim highlights the importance of these most fundamental core knowledge principles stating that:

> . . . at the roots of all our judgements there are a certain number of essential ideas which dominate all our intellectual life: they are what philosophers since Aristotle have called the 'Categories of Understanding': ideas of time, space, class, number, cause, substance, personality etc. They correspond to the most universal properties of things. They are like the solid frame which encloses all thought.
>
> (Durkheim, 1976, p.9)

Time is classified here as being among the most important 'categories of acknowledged understanding'. This is based on a common understanding of acknowledged facts and universal thought. From this anchorage point, sociologists and anthropologists have approached the study of time. Viewing the world from a socio-temporal perspective is central to this paper and is maintained for temporal explanation at the research site. As Sorokin states:

> . . . whereas the sociologists and social thinkers of the preceding periods thought of time, space, and causality as being quite simple, clear, uniform, and comprehensible as innate forms in our mind, the recent studies have shown that there are many different social times, different social spaces, different causalities even quite different forms and criteria of truth and of the methods of cognition especially of socio-cultural realities.
>
> (Sorokin, 1966, p.596)

Durkheim also asserts the social origins of time, adding to the sociological grounding of temporality, stating:

> . . . from the fact that the ideas of time, space, class, cause or personality are constructed out of social elements, it is not necessary to conclude that they are devoid of all objective value. On the contrary, their social origin rather leads to the belief that they are not without foundation in the nature of things.
>
> (Durkheim, 1976, p.19)

In industrial society, temporality in partially borne out of the notion that time is money and the idea that synchronisation of many people's timetables is important for industrial efficiency. That is why timekeeping becomes a moral issue. People late for work cost organisational efficiency, and with an agreement that one will supply blocks of contracted time then a failure to do so causes the organisations to introduce disciplinary proceedings. Another interesting observation of pre-industrial societies in this way is that time is not measured in fine detail. Hours, minutes and seconds have no currency and thus there is rarely urgency.

The social significance of clocks emerged from the 'fourteenth century onwards when church clocks and public clocks were erected in cities and large market towns' (Thompson, 1967, p.63). In terms of industrial society clocks and time become important with the introduction of a nationwide rail timetable that meant that two towns had to synchronise their clocks. Prior to this there was little necessity or relevance of time to life. Theorists comment importantly on the idea that it is the man who owns the timetable who owns time. As an instrument of order it is a powerful tool.

The demands of western society command that imposed temporal rhythms are complied with in the pursuit of industrial efficiency, productivity and communication. In the service industries that provide 24 hour delivery there is a temporal imposition that over-rides dominating temporal rhythm of the typical working day of nine-till-five (as far as working time is concerned). Antisocial shift working adds a competing temporal rhythm to the working week and illustrates the dominance of the work ethic as a temporal entity. For example, those who work shifts at Ashworth work to a daily sequence of, four on, two off, with unusual spans of duty (from 13.00–22.00 for two days; from 06.50–13.00 for another two days, two days off, then the cycle is repeated)

Temporal control

Time is an important resource to be effectively managed. Resources and efficiency are important to any business, and the NHS is no exception in the wake of a New Labour government, which has extended the combination of marketisation and managerialism inherited from the Conservative government in 1997, with its accompanying priorities, often bound in legislation and the dominance of the notion of efficiency of action. Of late that notion has further dominated as a doctrine with national policy initiatives like clinical governance (Scally and Donaldson, 1998). Time as a resource is controlled through organisationally owned timetables. These prescribed timetables further control temporality. As noted, 'time is becoming money, the employers' money' (Thompson, 1967, p.61), although even today the clock is unrivalled for work measurement in rural areas (piece work) to locate the quantity of work completed. The establishment of time as a social commodity is apparent from Marxist theory, with cyclicity of time being important to that organisational goal. Bock (1966) highlights the temporal power of the employer. Fundamentally, power in the realm of social time means the power to say 'do it now or else!' (Bock, 1966, p.98).

Introducing temporality and Ashworth

A socio-temporal conflict unfolds in the hospital setting also. There is the imposed temporal restraint of timetables and schedules with the accompanying routine, ritual and repetition necessary for smooth organisational operation. It is worth noting that, like children, the patients are timetabled to go to bed early, while patients, on the other hand have other priorities, particularly discharge as a basic value and a very important benchmark. Contextualising temporal frameworks is an important notion, as socio-temporal concepts often have meaning only in a given context. Zerubavel (1981, p.89) makes the point that 'the relevance of any unit of time depends on the particular cognitive context within which it is used'. For example, an academic trimester has no significance within a hospital setting, just as gaining a tribunal for an involuntary patient in a mental health facility has no temporal benchmarking quality in a university. Sick people do not fall ill to a schedule, so special arrangements are required to order temporal matters.

The meaning of local temporal order for organisations like Ashworth is reported on by both Roth (1963) and Zerubavel (1979), who have focused on organisational temporality and have to varying degrees offered explanations. They approach organisational temporality from different perspectives. Roth (1963) reports on hospital temporal order. He has at the nucleus of his argument the social significance of what he describes as 'temporal benchmarks' (Roth, 1963, p.14) which underscore the lack of relevance of the clock and the calendar. These have little cognitive importance, as different constructions of time and cadences dominate the specific organisational context. Sorokin and Merton (1937, p.621) reiterate this point at a more universal level, emphasising the general application of the concept that 'the system of time varies with the social structure'. Zerubavel (1979) focuses on the concept of cyclicity and the significance of repetition and preset rhythms for the sake of temporal order and temporal prediction in the hospital context.

The ownership of organisational temporality primarily manifests in the schedule or timetable (Zerubavel, 1981). It grounds sequencing, duration, location and frequency of occurrence. Notwithstanding cautions I made earlier about the literal transpositions of asylums, Ashworth Hospital is a typical total institution (Goffman, 1961). It has the accompanying timetables of collective activity, of collective duration, location and more often than not, frequency of occurrence. 'In the closed system people do not know their ages in years, but deduce their ages from their development' (Roth, 1963, p.97). In this site, 'development' is the health career. In short, Ashworth Hospital can be understood sociologically from a Durkheimian perspective.

As well as being organised through collective activity, so temporality is operated through a multiplicity of collectivities, realised through many concurrent time-tables. Further, its links with wider socio-temporality are more obscure than for other organisations, restating the social insularity that the Blom-Cooper Report noted (Blom-Cooper *et al.*, 1992). The social position of Ashworth with its isolation from society has similarities to tribal societies like those of the Inuit, the Tiv or the Kaguru. Because of this social quarantine the conditions are suitable for local time systems to develop and maintain themselves, particularly in a culture preoccupied with itself.

But it would be remiss to explore only theory relating to health care, when Ashworth Hospital is an amalgam. It is a hospital in many senses and a prison in others. It is certainly a prison as defined by the residents, who often prefer to be known as prisoners and on discharge will often use a prison sentence as a cover story to explain their long period away. So we progress to another sojourn to the relevant literature and a brief consideration of the social and temporal issues from this view

Prisoners, prisons and socio-cultural temporality

While a multitude of similarities exist between prison and hospital temporalities, prisons are fundamentally different from hospitals as far as the human commodities of their respective temporalities are concerned. Prison is primarily about serving time for a crime; hospital is supposed to be about a benevolent relationship of altruism as the recipient of care adopts a sick role. In prison the general principle is, the more severe the crime, the greater the length of time served, though treatments for mental disorders are available in prison with some penal institutions specialising in particular offence-related work (e.g. Grendon Prison and sex-offence work, Barlinnie Prison and therapeutic community work). An important benchmark as a prisoner is the EDR. Ashworth patients are without that important pre-determined benchmark that would officially recognise well-being or more importantly, denote discharge and liberty at the onset of detention, though there is a hidden benchmark of the average length of stay at 8.3 years.

While there are differences, there are many similarities. For example, staff and patients are both bound within a balanced, bargained order that maintains control in the hands of the authorities. For the staff who have the day-to-day, one-on-one contact with the detained criminal, 'the crimes of even the most serious offenders lose their significance with the passage of time' (Sykes 1971, p.55). This is a common feature at Ashworth and in the prison. The rationale for detention is less of a priority over time. Each patient disperses into the collectivity, a feature common to both prison and hospital environments.

Within a society there are many competing socio-temporal cycles that have changing significances depending on contextual and cognitive importance at any given point. It appears that the individual synchronises himself to conform to the order and relative dominance at any given point, and will generally operate accordingly. A failure to operate within these prior prescribed temporal responsibilities (particularly in prison) that bring about order and are bound with moral and ethical meanings, brings sanctions that are given in proportion to the broken temporal rhythm.

Sykes (1971) analyses a maximum-security prison sociologically. Ashworth is a closed social system similar to the focus of Sykes' work. He makes the point that 'serving time' is a relatively new concept that surfaced with the beginning of the 19th century, brought about by the growing trend of humanitarianism that meant it was more appealing than the physical punishments that had been used as sanctions previously:

> The philosophy of the enlightenment aided the belief that at long last society could make the punishment fit the crime by rationally assigning sentences of various lengths with the handy metric of time.
>
> (Sykes, 1971, p.XI)

Some feel that the onset of the industrial revolution was a catalyst that promoted incarceration and the accompanying cheap labour from the prisoner (e.g. prison labour was used to build Broadmoor Hospital and was tasked with other work), that in turn accompanied an acceleration of its popularity with central government. Carrell and Laing (1982) focus on the special unit in Barlinnie prison in Scotland, and quote from a prison diary similar sentiments that reflect a strong aspiration on the prisoners' behalf to control their own temporality.

> I rose at five thirty in the morning as normal and began my deep breathing exercises while waiting for the cell doors to be opened at six o'clock. I allowed my thoughts to wander freely in order to unwind the cobwebs. When the cell doors were opened I had my blankets folded and was ready to begin another day. I ran out to the yard and was immediately aware of the scent in the air coming from the flowers. It was the only point during the day that I was really free because I imagined most people were still asleep in the city.
>
> (Carrell and Laing, 1982, p.35)

Regardless of situation, compliance with contextually defined timetables, scheduling and routines as well as time investments are important, and again convey clear social messages. Non-compliance conveys moral messages and attracts sanctions. There is a collectivity to the temporal infrastructure of the ward that brings with it a socio-temporal order, with acquiescence preventing chaos, and dissent cast as deviance. Organisational ownership of communal temporal reference frameworks is important for the arrangements of daily life for large groups of people.

Next, socio-temporal concepts are explained more contextually, in terms of the ward. We can observe the impact of organisational timetables and other temporal influences on the trajectory of the individual. We have already alluded to the idea of, 'who owns the timetable' being a pivotal power issue equating to owning time. We now explore these key issues.

The socio-temporal world of the ward

Who owns time?

> The ward staff and the RMO [responsible medical officer] decide together with the Home Office I think. Nobody has ever said.
>
> (patient in participant observation)

In a situation where time is in abundance (with unlimited detention, time availability is in excess, unlike most situations where time is scarce) it appears incongruous to suggest there is a need for time creation. In this case patients talked of the need to generate time of their own, that they owned, and made clear distinctions about when they were free to use time as their own and when the organisation owned time, either through clinical timetables set for one ward or even one patient, or hospital-wide timetables. They saw creating their own time frame as a priority, using a variety of strategies, but the idea of who owns time can be seen in two rudimentary ways. Firstly, official documents reveal an organisational tricycle cadence revolving about the nursing shifts (arranged for organisational efficiency, as opposed to being needs led[4]). Secondly, the responses of those on the wards are exemplars of the common stock of knowledge on the wards in terms of this aspect of life, and reveal a common sense of perplexity on any trajectory towards discharge.

For example, patient responses to the question: 'Just when will you get out of here?' appeared cryptic and veiled, as if they did not want me to know the answer. 'It depends . . .', 'I am waiting for the Home Office . . . ', 'the care team decide . . .', 'who knows? . . .' were all responses from patient participants to this question.

Beyond this, it becomes further evident here that 'predicable rhythms' dominate the day and other cycles are apparent over longer periods. The day pulses in a trimester anchored around the nurses' shifts. Activities are punctured in the documentation into am, pm and night, the three shifts in any one day. The daily rhythm operates for maximum organisational efficiency whatever any clinical imperatives.

More 'deviant' patients will refuse to comply with this strategy of collective movement and will refuse to go to work, or in other cases resist leaving the ward in such circumstances.

It is in the official documentation that many examples of this cycle are evident and it is to these we turn to offer some explanations. The first is the 'movement ticket' that must accompany any patient off the ward. Most obviously the ticket is categorised into am, pm or night. The 'ward census report' is completed by each ward on a daily basis and details information about some basic aspects of the ward. It is an official account of the core daily activities. It is located within the metric of the clock and then the tricycle rhythm is used to collect data along the am, pm, night pattern. It is noticeable that as a native, one is not aware of these events or the language that accompanies them. It is only in the research that the temporal issues become obvious. The extent that time ownership is reinforced by the notion of a unique, taken-for-granted language of 'movements', and 'romeos' that accompany it is in the synchronising of all the wards to the hospital cadence and timetables. Ward nursing staff police time and timetables in a similar way to the traffic warden. As one patient stated: 'staff make sure we are where we should be all the time. They do spot checks, roll calls and use the work board, it's like a cattle run'.

Along with organisational timetables, the clinical trajectory can be estimated by the individual patient using social markers in hospital to mark off time to discharge. This is particularly problematic in a special hospital.

---

4   This is revealed simply as a little-recognised fact, common to organisational arrangements, not as a moral point.

Clinical time

The statements below give an alarming interpretation, given the patient is officially detained for treatment. However, patients often have little confident conception that a recovery will mean discharge. There is a sense that natural 'maturation' is generally the only route out, and irrespective of recovery one must serve time for the crime. Some quotes below highlight the situation as far as patients are concerned

> It doesn't matter if you get better. It doesn't mean you will get out of here.
>
> (patient in participant observation)

> I have been here for 19 years now. I only come for assessment. They promised me all sorts of treatment. All I have had is paracetamol, honestly.
>
> (patient in participant observation)

Clinical time does not extend to any sense of a discernable personal trajectory, though the periodicity to care teams marks an important local temporal cycle. Patients complain of a time 'vacuum', and use other similar phrases to carry the same meaning. 'Time warp' was commonly used by interviewees to express how they felt about time in a secure hospital, and is an oft-used term in participant observation. Patients complained of several reasons for this phenomenon including:

- no places available for them to progress
- their behaviour in the meantime has cancelled out plans
- a change of RMO or care team with different opinions
- a national policy change that excludes previous opportunity
- the patient has spoken of past events
- the patient has spoken about thoughts that are considered dangerous.

Patients fabricate pasts for other patients and create a forensic past more damning than their own. This is a particular feature for those who have sexually offended against children. Despite popular opinion, patients are not morally destitute, and many find crimes against children unacceptable.

Political cycles and time

Sometimes, more elementary and deep-seated temporal shifts are inflicted on the organisation as political imperatives cut across any previous temporal arrangements. This is exemplified by the patient statement:

> I was on track before the last inquiry.
>
> (patient in a focus group)

There is a marker that symbolises the beginning of a new temporal universe with most that has usually been important in temporal terms deconstructed, and a new order introduced. This new politically imposed order (negotiated with a gun held at the head of the bureaucracy) ultimately has implications for the length of detention, as the norms of forensic health care are redefined (through external inquiry). This manifests as a collective sense of temporal chaos. Most importantly this marker has been woven into the cultural fabric of Ashworth so that this periodic imbroglio is a climax, predicted like an earthquake reshuffling previous life and temporalities. 'We know it will happen, but we do not know when.'

The tutored observer can spot early signs – minor trembles – so cover can be sought but the course cannot be altered. Both patients and staff commonly refer to the next inquiry as this marker. A staff typifies this, stating, 'I'm bearing in mind the next inquiry, how it will look', another, 'I keep my head down. It's OK now but this will be the next inquiry. I want nothing to do with it'. A patient refers to the last inquiry, saying 'I was on track before the last inquiry. They stopped my LOAs [leaves of absence] and I am going backwards'. Another patient, unhappy with a personal situation says, 'wait until the next inquiry, my fuckin' MP knows what is going on and there are things happening outside this place'. He is engaging with the phenomenon and attempting to alter the course of Ashworth and his destiny by involving higher authorities.

Time warp: isolation and socio-temporality

> It's like a movie set. I'm sure the Home Office control even the weather. Go outside the wall and the weather is different.
>
> (patient in a focus group)

The insignificance of the clock and calendar has been noted, but patients explain time also as a vacuum. It is an empty expanse that they feel they need to fill. In this unstable socio-temporal arrangement, they appear to abandon any estimation as false hope, and enter enduring time whereby they surrender any estimation of how close they are to their discharge. This is what they describe as a vacuum. The cycles maintain themselves as a heartbeat does in a comatose patient, but they disengage with any sense of being in control of their own destiny. The meaning of time as control here is powerful. As the major commodity of a hospital detaining people for long periods of time, time manifests as a tool for implicitly punishing patients as 'unending time' is administered. Here, there is no foreseeable change and patients complain that they are not in a position to influence change. The incalculable notion of time to discharge adds to the idea that a 'time vacuum' exists at Ashworth. It is complicated by the idea that a clinical logic does not equate to detention ending. Patients detect what they term 'bullshit', denoting misinformation.

In wider society the annual cycles are religiously held (Christmas, Easter, Passover etc), with the financial imperatives (the business year, opening hours and work cycles) and educational terms among others. Few of us benchmark our days to the mental health review tribunals' case conferences, Mental Health Act Commission visits and canteen days that are at the core of local temporal benchmarks.

Local time reckoning

Canteen day is the most important day.
(patient in interview)

Local time reckoning is a common yet rarely recognised occurrence:

I'll see you on my next late.
(a nurse in participant observation)

Local time reckoning locates itself in local cycles, meanings and an estimated trajectory. Local time reckoning similar to the examples of isolated tribal societies emerges. The most obvious local estimates of time are the competing temporal cycles. The days are all segmented off into morning, afternoon and night, reinforced by the organisational rhythm of the shift patterns. Thereafter, the local cycles within a day are enshrined into the pattern of morning, afternoon and night for economic efficiency, having temporal patterns that fit neatly into the shift patterns as opposed to meeting individual need.

Subsequently, the official documentation augments the pattern so that the official recording follows again, the most dominant cycles. Patients and staff construct the day in such a way and use other metaphors to explain the notion including: am or pm, 'lates' and 'earlies'. The patients operate through shifts also. Their day is split in the same way. Events follow the same pattern, simply because the staff need to be around for a planned event to take place.

Time is estimated through the 'socials'. Socials are regular events, whereby patients in different wards go via a 'movement' to one central hall. These events are a major source of intelligence for patients that staff are not privy to. Illicit information is passed, as are goods including, on occasion, drugs. One patient told me in interview, 'you haven't got a clue what goes on in those socials . . . we know more than you do'. This is supported by nursing staff on the wards who often claim that if you want to know anything 'ask a patient'.

There is a code of silence on some issues at Ashworth that is supported by the need for confidentiality. This extends to a whole array of information. It is most accurate to state that, in general, patients are told what they need to know. Despite this and the communication restrictions, their intelligence is superior to that of the organisation. The social significance extends beyond the superficial to an important means of discovering. On the other hand, patients mark time and estimate time from these events. 'I'll see you at the next social', 'it was at the social when . . .' are common time estimators that make sense on one side of a 30-foot wall, but would be meaningless on the other.

You need to be careful. I have worked out that if they say 'six months', it means about 18 months, that's how things work in here, it's very slow.

Time, in here, it's so slow.

There is no timescale, they just say it will happen, nobody knows.

The Home Office, they decide. When they think I'm right I will move, it doesn't matter what you or anyone else thinks in here.

Several socio-temporal issues emerge here. The most obvious is the central importance of how the ward is organised. The next is the rigidity of the organisation, and the final point is the importance of maintaining oneself to the collective sequence. This is not only for oneself but for the maintenance of the sequencing order for the other patients. Paradoxically, if a patient becomes an expert sequencer and conveys his expectations when ward nursing staff do not comply, an illness label is attached and this behaviour is rationalised professionally as institutional neurosis or institutionalisation. Time-order compliance is converted to illness through the psychiatric frame of reference.

Paying with time for the crime

> You're all kidding yourselves.
>
> (patient in a focus group)

Patients commonly explain the detention as 'bird' or 'time'. This prison argot cements their common view that they are criminals paying for the crime. They see themselves as more appropriately dealt with under the criminal justice and penal systems as lawbreakers. Several pragmatic arguments reinforce their view. Patients often consider themselves as not being sick and therefore not requiring a hospital. They are also aware, through experience, that:

- treatment is often not available
- the length of stay begins as unclear and remains unclear
- detention can depend on many variables
- the judgment of the professionals can vary
- political fluctuations can alter length of stay
- sickness is not the only variable responsible for detention.

The patient respondents pointed out a 'mass delusion'. Here is an example:

> This is a fuckin' charade, everyone is going around pretending this is a hospital. What about the walls and the keys? What about treatment? Don't make me laugh.

On its own this could be the demented rambling of someone who is bitter with the system that detains. But he or she is detained as a patient and those others belonging to the ward then agree.

Methods of escaping time, and strategies to master time

> Get yourself a job on the ward, your time is your own then.
>
> (patient in a focus group)

Some patients would become a 'ward worker'. There are limited spaces on the wards and some wards do not have them. But they include 'kitchen man', 'stores', and occasionally 'laundry'. The exact role would start off clear to all the ward staff but become vague over time. The staff would end up referring to the patient and asking him or her about the role. This was the best example of mastery. The patient was able to go further than any other patient in space or time, circumventing official timetables. They would make requests to go to their room to get something essential to the role and wander about the ward almost unquestioned; they were perceived as doing the staff a favour and would gain other temporal 'gifts' as a result. They gained an expertise in the timetable of their own unique ward role and were able to command it to the extent of reprimanding staff for any non-compliance.

> I sleep. When you're asleep time just disappears.
>
> (patient in a focus group)

Paradoxically, sleep is heavily relied upon to cast away hours and days. If there was no planned activity patients would sleep where they could. Even when a planned activity was happening, patients could be seen sleeping. Their ability to find a remotely comfortable position was remarkable. Chairs were mostly preferred when the bed was not available. A coat has a multitude of roles. It can be rolled up into a pillow. It can be used as a mask to cut out light, or more conventionally when the hood is brought up to cover the face. Some patients sleep in a bolt upright position, appearing to be awake and so not drawing attention from nurses who are supposed to wake them up (waking patients up is to maintain sleeping patterns, considered to be important to maintain a healthy mental state). Spending one's own free time asleep helps, patients claim, to get rid of it:

> You go to sleep and like magic another three, four, five hours has gone, it's great. It means you are that much closer to getting out of here.

Patients also have remarkable strategies to manipulate time because of an excess of time, though they do not own most of it. Typically these include watching television, particularly 'soap'-type programmes, that are a constant interest. Television soap programmes are markers of calendar days.

The sick role

> I can't go to the workshops today, I'm sick.
>
> (patient in interview)

Time mastery was the deviant activity from a psychiatrised point of view, interpreted as non-compliance. For patients, it appeared to be an essential part of their survival. Whereas most patients could not estimate how long they would be detained they did quickly gain the skills of at least some temporal mastery. Much to the annoyance of nursing staff they would claim a physical illness, a headache, a stomach ache or diarrhoea. They were rarely if ever required to produce evidence. This would result in them 'staying off work'. This meant they had some charge over their timetable and thus some mastery.

The role of the television

The typical ward has several communal televisions that are used every day by at least some of the patients. Additionally, most patients have their own TV and video recorder that they use in the privacy of their own room. The TV has a role of consuming time, not unlike the role it has in homes up and down the country. However, it has a different significance. In participant observation I noticed several aspects to the use of the communal TV. The first was when there was an important social event to be screened. Wimbledon, European football, the rugby world cup and so on. Ward staff would gift 'time off' from workshops and alter the daily timetable (this was easier because patients did not go to work and so there was no need to synchronise the ward activities to the rest of the hospital). The TV would be watched by most people on the ward with the charge nurse and sometimes the ward manager taking a prime seat.

The TV was heavily relied on by the patients for the news of the outside world. It was their main contact with the outside world and with ecological time in the absence of any participation in the social life of the external environment that they observed in small portions throughout the day. In part, they gathered their knowledge about the world beyond the ward from this source. They would frequently ask questions about the meaning of news for them, and I deduced their concerns about their futures in some of these questions. This would most often become apparent when an individual would question their ability to survive in the world observed on the TV news. This appeared to become more of a concern with the passage of detention. The newspapers were also an obvious alternative, and the ward newspapers attracted the same level of interest.

Conclusions

This chapter has introduced concepts into forensic mental health work that were previously not debated. It has also addressed old issues from the world view of the 'little man', of those who live or work on the ward. This chapter stands as a blasphemous new theory set against the pseudo-religious clinical argot of 'care pathways' and 'dependencies' etc. From the pure clinical world view, I acknowledge there is equal truth, not as is claimed to be, the only truth. I hope the reflective discourse of clinical truth is not just a mantra and is able to accommodate these new theories.

It follows that while the 'little man' does not concur with official classifications and has his own taxonomies, he cannot generally comprehend his own trajectory from admission to discharge. Temporality appears to be grounded in the official master timetables, but there are a number of strategies employed by patients to master their own time. Markers of progress were not apparent and patients described a temporal vacuum. Patients developed a variety of strategies to master time, but these could be interpreted morally and psychiatrically.

Local time reckoning is observed in a tricycle day and other emergent social markers of time, marking off various periodicities (e.g. canteen day, socials, tribunals, and patient care team meetings). The four- and six-day week compete with the seven-day week. The nine-till-five day has only minimal significance. This temporal chaos must lead to implications for both the Mental Health Act

(1983) and for national policy. It cannot be reasonable to detain people in a temporal vacuum under the pretext of health care.

It also seems unacceptable to be able to detain anyone without limit of time to deliver treatment and not be bound into a contract to honour that promise. It should not be acceptable to use the broadest definitions of 'therapy' to claim that meaningful treatment for a patient's particular problems is occurring. Cookery, joinery and swimming as therapies for a rapist have never been effective. Assessing him years into detention for treatment seems to be a sinister use of health care for social control.

Patients were not able to demonstrate a 'career' or trajectory from admission through to discharge. Significant markers, usually taken from the social situation, of progress through this passage were not observable. Patients would describe being in a temporal 'vacuum', without a date for release or any reliable social markers of time to assess any 'journey' towards discharge (the most important goal of most patients). A lack of treatment is concealed through definitional inter-pretations. The organisation defines any activity as treatment. Those on the wards are more specific and do not include entertainment, activities that draw on a work ethic (joinery, metalwork, etc) or education as treatment. Neither do patients and staff refer to detention as treatment (the Mental Health Act provides that for some patients detention prevents deterioration). With changes afoot in British mental health legislation, this point about the conflation of mere deten-tion with treatment may become more and more a point of contention about human rights.

Staff on the wards are able to demonstrate a career towards their version of dis-charge. Retirement dates were frequently regaled. Staff would often be able to accurately estimate when they would be able to retire and could be very specific estimating up to 10 and even 15 years hence the day they would be able to leave (including holidays).

Patients skilfully use a variety of time disposal and creation techniques. These are used to extend a very limited ability to master some time for themselves outside of official timetables.

A tricycle day regulates the daily practice. This thrice-daily cycle reflects the shift system of the ward staff. All ward timetables studied used this template and each ward synchronised itself to this pattern that organised each ward. Each indi-vidual has a burden of functioning within this temporal framework, avoiding conflict. This temporal order, administered through timetables was inextricably tied to this local temporal pulse.

The 'tricycle day' is taken for granted, involving themes common to the arrangements of all the wards. First, that compliance to the common timetable is not negotiable and is a pivotal to social order. Secondly these common temporal markers throughout the day emerge as trilogies. Mealtime, medication rounds, shift start and finishes, begin and end each individual pulse in the day. This is predictable time through routinised local time reckoning, replacing the wider sense of a day with a 24-hour period split into three.

Participants (both patients and staff) have been conditioned on the special hos-pital wards to be subservient and allow 'outsiders' who we believe do not really comprehend the wards, to explain their dynamics. These interpretations have dominated, while those on the wards have remained obedient and silent. Keeping silent to these 'outside' interpretations, is considered by myself as a

Darwinian-type response to explanations that claim moral superiority, the 'truth' and foreclosure. It is with this backdrop and this thesis that the rest of the chapter is set.

The Mental Health Act (1983) does not currently impose any temporal deadlines for most detained patients at Ashworth. Neither does the Act impose any obligation to identify any dangerousness or individual risk issues. It therefore does not require that the prime reason for detention (dangerous, violent or criminal propensities) be explicitly addressed. Altering the Act to explicitly require statements of risk, the interventions required to effect change to risk and what criteria the patient would be required to achieve to gain discharge would help. Binding contracts for each individual's care should be enforced, and detention should continue until the risk is diminished. Penalties should be in place when relevant treatment is not delivered. Organisations have a duty to function effectively and efficiently. The organisation should be honest about its motivations and functions.

The Act should be mindful of the temporal experience, and therefore its code of practice should include the following:

1   explicit markers of achievement towards discharge (utilising local social markers as opposed to the clock)
2   the organisation's performance should be measured against these variables
3   the views of those on the wards should be included as a significant variable of the experienced, social situation
4   audits, star ratings and standards (that have gained the status of hyper-real) should be replaced by explanations by those on the wards of their own experience
5   further research of social variables should be a prerequisite to practice
6   the traditional organisation chart should be abandoned in favour of an upturned chart to reflect the areas of patient activity and address the social divisions expressed by those on the wards.

Any organisation that is responsible for the detention of people for periods measured in years and decades without any discernable endpoint should be cognisant of temporal issues. A central commodity of Ashworth is 'time', yet there is no realisation of the role time has at any level other than in terms of a particular illness experience. Awareness of temporality is a glaring omission for such an organisation.

Patients should be afforded a discernable future that is estimable. The need to be able to assess one's trajectory through time is a basic human need. This requires synthetic but recognisable 'temporal markers' that point out the journey to discharge. This is especially important where there is little reliability in assessing who one's peers really are.

The organisation should acknowledge its domination in temporal control. Each person on the ward, and in turn each ward, is synchronised to a common timetable owned by the organisation and the subject of intense surveillance in its many forms.

Local time reckoning on the wards replaces wider temporal ordering events. The social, the canteen and the MHRT are basic cycles of events that mark out various social punctuations in the passage of time. Additionally, there are competing 'weeks' in co-existence. The seven-day week is important for its punctuation by canteen and the slowed-down period of the 'weekend'. However, other periods are important. The four-day week is almost completely social in orientation and marks the period in which a social cycle is complete. It is followed by a two-day break – a 'weekend'. The three-day week also has a similar tempo and both coincide with the periods of 'shifts' worked by ward-based nurses. The previously described 'tricycle' day is a feature on every ward with its peculiar feature of a thrice-daily temporal pulse.

Patients require access to their own clinical notes to enable patients to assess their own trajectory through time by locating at least themselves in their own, psychiatrically owned clinical trajectory. Further research is required. This chapter examines time and the social experience on the wards. Other temporal perspectives and other cultural views should be sought.

References

Blom-Cooper L, Brown M, Dolan R and Murphy E (1992) *Report of the Committee of Inquiry into Complaints about Ashworth Hospital*. Cm 2028. London: HMSO.

Bock PK (1966) Social time and institutional conflict. *Human Organization* **2**: 96–102.

Carrell C and Laing J (1982) *The Special Unit, Barlinnie Prison: its evolution through its art: an anthology of essays, statements, art works, creative writings and documentary photographs*. Glasgow: Third Eye Centre.

Davies CA (1999) *Reflexive Ethnography: a guide to researching selves and others (ASA research methods in social anthropology)* London: Routledge.

Durkheim E (1976) *The Elementary Forms of Religious Life*. London: George Allen and Unwin.

Fallon P, Bluglass R, Edwards B and Daniels G (1999) *Report of the Committee of Inquiry into the Personality Disorder Unit, Ashworth Special Hospital*. Cm 4194. London: HMSO.

Goffman E (1961) *Asylums. Essays on the social situation of mental patients and other inmates*. Harmondsworth: Penguin.

Gouldner AW (1954) *Patterns of Industrial Bureaucracy*. New York: The Free Press.

Gurvitch G (1964) *The Spectrum of Social Time*. Dordrecht-Holland: D Reidel Publishing Company.

Moore WE (1963) *Man, Time and Society*. London: John Wiley and Sons Inc.

Pink Floyd (1974) Time. From: *The Dark Side of the Moon*. London: Harvest Records.

Roth J (1963) *Timetables: structuring the passage of time in hospital treatment and other careers*. New York: Bobbs-Merrill.

Scally G and Donaldson LJ (1998) Clinical governance and the drive for quality improvement in the new NHS in England. *British Medical Journal* **4 July**: 61–5.

Sorokin PA (1966) *Sociological Theories of Today*. London: Harper and Row.

Sorokin PA and Merton RK (1937) Social time: a methodological and functional analysis. *American Journal of Sociology* **426**: 15–29.

Sykes GM (1971) *The Society of Captives: a study of a maximum security prison*. Princeton: Princeton University Press.

Taylor C and White S (2000) *Practising Reflexivity in Health and Welfare: making knowledge*. Buckingham: Open University Press.

Thompson EP (1967) Time, work, discipline and industrial capitalism. *Past and Present* **37**: 57–97.

Waite T (1993) *Taken on Trust*. London: Hodder and Stoughton.

Zerubavel E (1979) *Patterns in Hospital Life*. Chicago: Chicago University Press.

Zerubavel E (1981) *Hidden Rhythms. Schedules and calendars in social life*. Chicago: Chicago University Press.

Index

Abramson, M   13
ACPAS *see* Ashworth CAB Patients'
    Advocacy Service
activity schedules   29, 46, 87–8, 146, 153
    see also time and temporality
Adshead, G   130
advocacy   81–4
  in secure environments   83–4, 91–4
    and confidentiality   82–3
Aitken, G and Jellicoe-Jones, L   109
Aitken, G and Logan, C   110
Aitken, G and Nobel, K   98
Aitken, G *et al*   109
Allan, K and Cawthorne, C   74
Allderidge, P   3
'anti-therapeutic' cultures   1
antisocial personality disorder, and
    dangerousness   18
Armstrong, S   14
Arnold ward (Ashworth)   44–50
  critical incident analysis   48
  daily activities   45, 46
Ashworth
  background history   3–5
    formation and early remits   5–6
    merger problems   28–30, 42–3
  culture and ethos   35–8
    and 'dangerousness'   16–18, 84
    and 'evil'   35–6
    and paranoia   129–31
    medicalisation processes   36
  environment and location   5, 86–7
  funding issues   54–5
  impact of 'scandal hospital' inquiries
      6–10, 52–5, 81–2, 139
    calls for closure   7–8
    delayed patient discharges   147–8
    introduction of advocacy   81–94
    introduction of consultants and task
        forces   53–5
    introduction of ward managers   53–5
    'pendulum effects'   8, 29–30
  management reorganisations   8, 32–3,
      52–5
    and therapeutic focus   33

media interest   7, 43
myths and narratives   24–6, 40
patient populations   2, 84–6
philosophical basis   35–6
public relations management   70–1
research studies   39–56
routines and activities   29, 46, 87–8,
    146, 153
socio-political contexts   11–16, 147–8
  governance of 'dangerousness'
      16–18
specific wards
  Arnold ward   44–50
  Blake ward   44–7
  Forster ward (young personality
      disorders)   48, 50–2
  Lawrence ward   93
  Owen ward   92–3
  Tennyson (admissions)   48, 49–50
temporal dimensions   143–55
training resources   69–70
see also Ashworth Women's Service
    (AWS)
Ashworth CAB Patients' Advocacy Service
    (ACPAS)   83–4, 89, 91–4
Ashworth Patients' Council   88–92
Ashworth Women's Forum   126–7
Ashworth Women's Service (AWS)
    97–115, 119–33
  demonisation and stigma issues
      119–20
  existing psychological input   100
  introducing enhanced psychological
      services   99–105
    resistance to change   105–9
  national policies and guidance   98–9
  personal motivations for working
      97–9, 119–21, 131–3
  service closure   109–13
Asylums (Goffman)   24, 39, 44, 49, 138–9

Baker, E   15
Bamber, Cary   12
Barlinnie prison (Scotland)   145
Barnes, DK   82–3

Beales, D   8
Bean, P   14–15
Benn, A and Laithwaite, H   74
Bentall, R and Haddock, G   74
Bethlem Hospital (London)   3
black and ethnic minority patients   85
Blackwood, Orville   7
Blake Ward (Ashworth)   44–7
  critical incident analysis   48
  daily activities   45, 46
Blankstein, H   18
Blom-Cooper Inquiry – 1992   7–9, 29,
    40, 81–2
  errors   54
  impact and effects   52–5, 81–2
  key recommendations   53
    on advocacy   81–2
  positive aspects   59
Bluglass, R   10
Boateng, Paul   89
Bock, PK   143
Bondi, L and Burman, E   100
Bowden, P   14
Boynton Report – 1980   6, 43
Boynton, J   5
Brady, Ian   43
Broadmoor
  background history   3–5
  critical reports   6–7
  patient deaths   6–7
Broverman, IK et al   132
Bustillo, J et al   72
Butler Committee – 1975 11, 13
Butterworth Report – 1994   62

Caldwell, G and Naismith, C   48
'care vs. control' discourses   11–18
Carrell, C and Laing, J   145
Carstairs High Security Hospital (Scotland)
    72, 74
Carton, Gerry   74
Caudill, W   46–7
Channel 4 documentaries   81
Chapman, P and McKeown, M   65
Cheadle Royal Psychiatric Hospital   39–40
  see also Elizabeth Campbell (EC) School
Chesler, P   129
Citizens Advice Bureau Patients Advocacy
    Service (ACPAS)   81–4
coercive/policing powers   15–16
  attitudes of psychiatrists   15–16
cognitive-behavioural therapies   59
  see also psychosocial interventions (PSI)
confidentiality issues

and advocacy work   82–3
and communication restrictions   149
and psychological services   105–7
  see also whistleblowing
consultancy firms   53–5
'convict's code' (Wieder)   51
'correction vs. prevention' debates   11–16
  key points of controversy   16–18
Corrigan, P and McCracken, S   61
Corrigan, P et al   61
'corruption of care' (Martin)   5–6, 12
'critical incidents'   39, 44
  Owen Ward   92–3
Cultural Awareness Group (CAG)   85
culture of Ashworth   35–8
  background history
    merger problems   28–30
    mid-1980s   1–3, 28–9
  and 'dangerousness'   16–18, 84
  and 'evil'   35–6
  and paranoia   129–31
    perpetuating mechanisms   24–6, 84
    safeguarding activities   70–1
  see also ward cultures
Cutting Edge documentary (Channel 4
    1991)   7, 81

Dachelet, CZ et al   39
daily routines   87–8, 146, 153
  see also time and temporality
dangerous and severe personality disorder
    (DSPD)   16
'dangerousness'
  governance discourses   16–18
  meanings and constructs   17
  see also paranoia at Ashworth; violence
Davies, CA   136
delayed discharges   85, 150
detention systems
  background history   4
  socio-political influences   152–3, 154
  see also 'correction vs. prevention'
    debates
discharges see patient discharges; patient
    transfers
dispersed regional units   10–11
'disturbed' patients   44–6
Dolan, R   99, 109
Douglas, D   55
Durkheim, E   141–2

Edge, D   110
education facilities (patients)   87–8
  see also staff training

Edwards, S   127
Elizabeth Campbell (EC) School   41–2
Elliot, G   56
Emerson, RM and Pollner, M   16
emotional expression issues
  research studies   72–3
  in women's services   127–9
environment and facilities   5, 86–7
ethnographic studies *see* research at
    Ashworth
Evans-Pritchard, EE   47
'evil', concepts and denials   35–6
Ewers, P *et al*   73, 74
expertise   31
  and experience   24
expressed emotion studies, staff—patients
    72–3
Exworthy, T and Gunn, J   8

Fadden, G   60
Fallon Inquiry – 1999   7, 8, 29, 72, 92–4,
    111
family interventions   68, 73
female patients
  daily activities   87
  history of detention   4
  policy mental health guidance   120–1,
      128
  status and position   132–3
  transfers   86, 109–11
    follow-ups   111–12, 115
  see also Ashworth Women's Service (AWS)
female staff   122–3
  emotional responses   128–9
  nurse students   42–3
Fennell, P   13
Fernando, S   100
Finnema, E *et al*   72–3
Fisherton House (Salisbury)   3
food and diet
  access to snacks   90
  consumption by staff   25
  cultural appropriateness   90
  effects of medication   90
'forensic institute' initiatives   33
Forster Ward (Ashworth)   48, 50–2
  contradictory discourses   52
Foster, J *et al*   73
Foucalt, M   36
funding issues   54–5

gallows humour   35
Geelan, S and Nickford, C   73
George, S   76

'ghosting' practices   92
Gillon, R   14
Glancy Report – 1974   11, 13
Goffman, E   24, 39, 44, 49, 138–9
Gouldner, AW   40, 139
Gournay, K and Sandford, T   60, 72
'governance of dangerousness'   16–18
group dynamics   12
group work, PDU female patients   123–6
'groupthink'   31
Gurvitch, G   141

halal meats   90
Hammond, PE   40
hate mail   1, 2
healthcare professionals *see individual
    professions*; staff at Ashworth
Hemmingway, C   98
Henry, J   47
Hiday, V   17
High Security Psychiatric Services
    Commissioning Board   9–10
  see also Special Hospital Service
      Authority (SHSA)
high-security hospitals *see* special hospitals
Hinshelwood, RD and Skogstad, W   130
historical perspectives
  of asylum and segregation   3–5
  of 'correction vs. prevention'   11–16
Holmes, D and Federman, C   36
'hope' and pessimism   36–8
Hospital Advisory Service *see* NHS Hospital
    Advisory Service (HAS) reports
Hospitals in Trouble (Martin 1984)   5–6
hostage taking incidents   93
humour   35
Hunter, C   50
Huxley, N *et al*   72

incidents *see* 'critical incidents'
induction sessions   43–4, 84, 121–2
Ingleby, D   15
inquiries and official reports   6–10, 52–5,
    81–2, 139
  Blom-Cooper Inquiry – 1992   7–9, 29,
      40, 81–2
  Fallon Inquiry – 1999   7, 8, 29, 72,
      92–4, 111
  impacts
    calls for closure   7–8
    delayed patient discharges   147–8
    introduction of advocacy   81–94
    introduction of consultants and task
        forces   53–5

inquiries and official reports – *contd*
  impacts – *contd*
    introduction of ward managers 53–5
    'pendulum effects' 8, 29–30
institutional systemic problems 5–6
  see also culture of Ashworth
Into the Mainstream (Department of Health
  2002) 120–1, 128
Isherwood, T *et al* 72
isolation factors 5–6

Jennings, A 127
Jones, L and Aitken, G 99
Jubb, M and Shanley, E 73

Kaye, Charles 9, 89
Kaye, C and Franey, A 8–9
Kean, B 30, 35
Koestler Awards 91
Kuipers, E 72

La Caze, M 36
Laithwaite, H 74
Lart, R *et al* 99
Lawrence Ward (Ashworth) 93
learning disabilities 2
  early legislation 4
Lee, D and Newby, H 23
Lees, GD *et al* 43
Leff, J 60
legislation, background history 3–4
Leibling, H 98
Link, B and Steuve, A 73
literature searches, ward cultures 47
Lofland, LH 44

McCann, E 72
McCann, G 59, 66, 77
McCann, G and McKeown, M 62, 66
McGuire, J 17, 59
MacInnes, D 73
McKeown, M and Liebling, H 71
McKeown, M and Stowell-Smith, M 36,
  70, 76
McKeown, M *et al* 60
Mahon, Alice 93
management of special hospitals 9
  changes and reorganisations 32–3, 52–5
Manning, N 16
Martin, JP 5–6, 12, 52
Martin, Michael 6
Mason, T and Mercer, D 24, 36
Mason, T *et al* 36
media interest 7, 43

and management practices 70–1
medicalisation of 'evil' 36
'medium-security' establishments 13
  see also regional secure units (RSUs)
Mental Deficiency Act – 1913 4
Mental Health Act – 1959 4, 14
Mental Health Act – 1983, and detention
  periods 152–3, 154
mental health review tribunals (MHRTs)
  138
Mercer, D and Richman, J 47
Mill, JS 14–15
Miller, G and Hood, R 37–8
MIND 9, 82
Mitchell, J 129
models of care (nursing) 31
Monahan, J 13
Moore, E *et al* 73
Moore, WE 141
Moos, R and Hoots, P 47
Moran, T and Mason, T 34
Morgan, G 30–1
Moss Side
  history 4
  location 5
  merger problems 28–30
  patient profiles 5
  see also Ashworth
myths and rumours 40

narratives and story-telling 24–6
new staff
  induction procedures 84
  sabotage strategies 53
  and 'story-telling' 25–6
newspaper reading 152
NHS Hospital Advisory Service (HAS)
  reports 6–7, 8
nurses
  attitudes towards other professionals
    48
  attitudes towards patients 1, 8, 45–6,
    122–3
  impact of reorganisations 32–3
  students 42–3
nursing cultures *see* ward cultures

O'Carroll, M *et al* 60
O'Donoghue, EG 3
OER (education department) 87–8
Offe, C 5
Olesen, V 40, 55–6
open hospitals, acute units, conditions 11
organisations, as 'psychic prisons' 30–1

Owen Ward (Ashworth)   92–4

paedophile rings   29, 92, 93
paranoia at Ashworth   129–31
   perpetuating mechanisms   24–6, 84
   safeguarding activities   70–1
   see also 'dangerousness'
Park Lane   5
   culture   26
   merger problems   28–30
      studies   42–3
   opening   5, 26–7
   procedures and policies   26–7
Parker, E   3–4
Parkhurst Prison   4
Parry-Crooke, G   98, 100, 123
paternalism   14–15
patient councils   88–91
Patient Days magazine   88–9, 90–1
patient deaths, at Broadmoor   6–7
patient discharges
   delayed   85, 150
   impact of inquiries   147–8
patient history presentations   48
patient transfers   85–6
   females   109–12, 115
patients
   attitudes towards each other   45–6
   attitudes towards therapy   52
   attitudes towards time   143–52
   general characteristics   2, 84–6
   impact of interventions   30
   length of stay   85, 144–8, 150, 154
   personality disorders   18, 50–2
   psychotic or disturbed   44–6, 73–4
   'role' in hospitals   46
PDU (personality disorder unit)   91–3
   female patients   123–9
   see also Forster ward (Ashworth)
'pendulum effect' (libertarian–
   authoritarian reactions)   8, 29–30
personality disorders
   and 'dangerousness'   18
   facilities at Ashworth   50–2, 91–2
      and advocacy services   91–3
      and moral reasoning   51
   see also dangerous and severe personality
      disorder (DSPD); PDU (personality
      disorder unit)
pharmacological interventions   14
Pidd, F   109
Pilgrim, D   1, 15–17
Pilgrim, D and Eisenberg, N   1, 114
Pilgrim, D and Rogers, A   15, 18

Pink Floyd   137
policing/coercive powers   15–16
   attitudes of psychiatrists   15–16
Pollner, M and Emerson, RM   44
Potier, M   120, 127
Powell, Enoch   10–11
Prison Officers' Association (POA)
   culture and ethos   1, 41–2
   influence   41–2, 43
prisons, and prevention   13–14
prn medication, and patient deaths   6–7
psychiatric profession
   attitudes to coercion   15
   role in special hospitals   30–1
'psychic prisons'   30–1
psychological interventions (women's
      services)   97–115
   group work   123–6
   mission statement   104
   personal accounts and motivations
      97–9, 119–21
   proposed changes   99–100
      implementing changes   102–5
      recruiting and developing the team
         103–5
   record keeping   104
   resistance to changes   105–9
      competency concerns   105–7
      confidentiality issues   105–7
      'safeguarding' patients   107–8
      team concerns   108–9
   review processes   104–5
   staff disbanding arrangements   112–13
   see also psychosocial interventions (PSI)
psychosis, and psychosocial interventions
      73–4
psychosocial interventions (PSI)   59–77
   approaches   60–1
   evidence base   62–3, 64, 72–4
   proposed introduction to Ashworth
      61–5
      models and approaches   63
      and staff training   63–5
   resistance to initial proposals   65–72
      financial concerns   67
      lack of knowledge   67–9
      organisational impediments   66–7
   recent developments at Ashworth
      76–7
public inquiries *see* inquiries and official
      reports
public relations management   70–1

Radzinowicz, L and Hood, R   17

Rae, Malcolm   54
Rampton
   history   4
   mistreatment of patients   5
      Boynton Report – 1980   6, 43
   patient profiles   4
Rapoport, R   8
Rask, M and Levander, S   72–3
'Rebecca Myths' (Gouldner)   40
recruitment, psychological services   103
Reed review   62
reflexivity   23
regional secure units (RSUs)   11
research at Ashworth
   comparative literature searches   47
   personal accounts and reflections
      39–56
      background and impetus   39–44
      dissemination of findings   47–8
      feedback workshop sessions   40,
         47–8
      outcomes of reports   48–50
   staff resignations   33
restraint measures, and patient deaths
   6–7
Richman, J   31, 40, 42
Richman, J and Mason, T   24, 40
Richman, J and Mercer, D   53–4
Richman, J et al   55
risk assessments
   of the institution   14
   of patients   12–13, 17–18
risk management   17–18
Ritchie Report – 1984   6
Rogers, A and Pilgrim, D   3, 5, 8
Romme, M et al   65
Rosenhan, DL   47
Ross, R and Fabiano, E   59
Ross, R and Gendreau, P   59
Roth, J   141, 143
RSUs see regional secure units
rumours and myths   40
   see also narratives and story-telling

Scally, G and Donaldson, LJ   142
Scott, PD   13
Scott, S and Williams, J   99
Scull, A   10, 15
Secret Hospital (Yorkshire Television)   6, 43
security concerns, reports and inquiries
   7–8
security training   43–4, 84, 121–2
sex offenders, treatment concepts   14
Shaw, J et al   99, 109

Shooter, Mike   15
shop facilities   89–90
Showalter, E   127
SHSA see Special Hospital Service
   Authority
sick roles   151
sleep and time   151
smoking activities   45, 48, 90
social events   149
'social therapy' initiatives   33
socio-temporal theories   140–3
Sociologists at Work (Hammond)   40
solitary confinement   7
Sorokin, PA   141
Sorokin, PA and Merton, RK   141, 143
A Special Hospital (Channel 4 1991)   7, 81
Special Hospital Service Authority (SHSA)
   critical reports   6–7
   leadership and management teams   9
   replacement authorities   9–10
   see also High Security Psychiatric Services
      Commissioning Board
special hospitals
   background history   3–5
   critical reports and inquiries   6–8
   detention systems   4
   patient deaths   6–7
   proposals for closure   8–10
   'therapy vs. detention' frameworks
      11–18
staff at Ashworth
   attitudes of external peers   31, 40, 139
   attitudes towards patients   1–2, 24,
      44–5
      emotional responses   128–9
      narratives and story-telling   24–6
   engaging in 'bad' behaviours   34–5
   impact of the organisation   2, 30–1
   problems with morale   32–3
   promotion systems   71
   supportive and compassionate   2, 71
   see also female staff; new staff
staff training
   in psychosocial interventions (PSI)
      63–5
   resources   69–70
staff-expressed emotion   128–9
   research studies   72–3
Stafford, P   123
Stanton, HA and Schwartz, MS   47
Steadman, HJ et al   18, 73
story-telling and narratives   24–6
stress-vulnerability model of care   63
student nurses   42–3

substance misuse, and dangerousness   18
Swanson, J et al   73
Swift, J   77
Sykes, GM   144–5
Szasz, TS   16, 17

Tarrier, N   60
Tarrier, N et al   74
task forces   53–5
tautologies   17
Taylor, C and White, S   136
Taylor, L and Jones, S   73
Taylor, P et al   73
television watching   152
temporal control   142–3
temporal knowledge   141–2
temporality see time and temporality
Tennyson Ward (Ashworth admissions)
    48, 49–50
Terkel, S   37
'therapeutic community principles'   92
therapeutic interventions
    barriers to implementation   61, 65–72,
        105–9
    concepts   138, 153
    efficacy   30
    innovation attempts   60
    patient attitudes towards   52
    see also psychological interventions
        (women's services); psychosocial
        interventions (PSI)
Thompson, EP   142–3
Thomson, L   72–3, 76
Thorn Diploma   60–6
Thrasher, J and Smith, HL   47
Tilt Report – 2000   7–8, 111
time and temporality   92, 140–55
    autobiographical relevance   135–8
    key theoretical perspectives   140–3
    recommendations   154–5
    socio-temporal aspects of Ashworth
        143–55
        clinical time   147
        escaping/mastering time   150–52
        isolation and time warps   148
        local time reckoning   149–50
        ownership issues   145–6
        paying for crime   150–1
        political time   147–8
    specific significance   140–1
training see education facilities (patients);
    staff training
transfers see patient transfers
transport facilities   90

treatments see therapeutic interventions
Trust Matters (newspaper)   139
TV documentaries   6–7, 81

user forums, women's services   126–7
Ussher, J   129, 133

Van Humbeeck, G et al   72
Van Maanen, J   39
violence
    causes   11–12, 17, 48
    and personality disorders   50
    risk predictors   17–18
    see also 'dangerousness'
Vishnick, C et al   74
Vivienne-Byrne, S   106
Von Economo, C   4

Waite, Terry   137–8
Walker, H   72, 74
Walker, H and Connaughton, J   74
ward cultures   1, 8, 28–9, 45–6
    literature searches   47
        anthropological models   47
    and 'models of care'   31
    research studies   39–56
    role of narrative   24–6
ward managers (WMs)   40, 53–5
    surveys   54–5
'ward workers'   150–1
Watts, Joseph   6–7
Webster, C   4
Wessley, S et al   73
Wheeler Report   41
whistleblowing   2, 35
    recriminations   84
Whittaker, D and Stickley, T   73
Wieder, DL   51
Williams, E et al   74
Williams, Dr Richard   89
Winter, R   23
WISH see Women in Secure Hospital
Women in Secure Hospital (WISH)   98,
    111
Women Working with Women   99
women's forum   126–7
women's services see Ashworth Women's
    Service (AWS)
Women's Strategic Development
    Guidance (Department of Health
    2002)   133
workshop facilities   87–8

Zerubavel, E   141, 143